D0080209

R. Scott Sullender, PhD

Losses in Later Life
A New Way of Walking with God
Second Edition

More pre-publication
REVIEWS, COMMENTARIES, EVALUATIONS . . .

"As I first looked at its table of contents, my initial reaction was that this book sounded awfully negative ('Grief,' 'Loss,' etc.). However, as I moved through the chapters, I became increasingly aware of how well the author was providing quite *positive* responses—both psychological and spiritual—to these very real experiences of loss.

I was struck with how well Sullender uses illustrations and case studies throughout to make his point clear and relevant. Reading from the perspective of later years, I found myself reflecting over and over again: 'Been there; done that!'

Sullender writes, of course, from the perspective of a counselor. As an adult educator, I became very aware of the degree to which his chapters could also provide the basis for a whole curriculum of adult learning experiences in the local church. Too much adult religion education starts at the point of doctrine—what the church wants to teach its people—instead of with issues in people's personal lives. This excellent book could trigger a companion volume exploring its implications for teaching ministries with adults.

Although primarily for practitioners, *Losses in Later Life* can also help those actually experiencing such personal losses to better understand how they truly are part of the reality of life."

Kenneth Stokes, PhD
Executive Director,
Adult Faith Resources,
Minneapolis, MN

The Haworth Pastoral Press
An Imprint of The Haworth Press, Inc.

Losses in Later Life
A New Way of Walking with God

Second Edition

Losses in Later Life
A New Way of Walking with God

Second Edition

R. Scott Sullender, PhD

The Haworth Pastoral Press
An Imprint of The Haworth Press, Inc.
New York • London • Oxford

Published by

The Haworth Pastoral Press, an imprint of The Haworth Press, Inc., 10 Alice Street, Binghamton, NY 13904-1580

Cover design by Monica L. Seifert.

Library of Congress Cataloging-in-Publication Data

Sullender, R. Scott.
　　Losses in later life : a new way of walking with God / R. Scott Sullender.—2nd ed.
　　　　p.　　cm.
　　Includes bibliographical references and index.
　　ISBN 0-7890-0628-6 (alk. paper).
　　1. Loss (Psychology) in old age. 2. Life change events in old age. 3. Adjustment (Psychology) in old age. 4. Aging—Psychological　aspects. 5. Aged—Psychology. 6. Aged—Religious life. 7. Aged—Pastoral counseling of. I. Title.
BF724.85.L67S85 1999
155.67—dc21　　　　　　　　　　　　　　　　　　　　　　　　　　　99-17250
　　　　　　　　　　　　　　　　　　　　　　　　　　　　　　　　　　　　CIP

CONTENTS

ABOUT THE AUTHOR

R. Scott Sullender, PhD, is Executive Director at the Samaritan Counseling Center, in Upland, California. He is also an ordained Presbyterian minister, a licensed psychologist in the state of California, and a Diplomate with the American Association of Pastoral Counselors. Dr. Sullender has twenty-five years of experience as a psychologist, pastor, chaplain, pastoral counselor, and administrator. He has written and lectured in the areas of loss and grief, aging and spirituality, and theology and personality. Dr. Sullender is the author of *Grief and Growth: Pastoral Resources for Emotional and Spiritual Growth; Losses in Later Life: A New Way of Walking with God;* a forthcoming book, *Passing Through: Reflections on the 23rd Psalm;* and numerous Christian educational curricula.

Preface

Life is a journey. There are many stages along the way. Most of these stages include loss experiences. We lose people we love through death, through divorce, through "growing apart." We can lose a job, a home, a pet, or a valued possession. We can also lose moments, ideals, dreams, and health. Some losses are sudden and very painful. Others come upon us more gradually and with mixed feelings. Either way losses are inevitable. They seem to be part and parcel of the nature of life itself. The terrible agony of an unwanted loss is as "natural" to life as is the joy of new birth, and in some cases, they are mysteriously linked.

The losses that occur during the first half of life are often couched in terms of growth and development. Losing our first tooth, graduating from school, and losing one's innocence are often understood as prerequisites for growth. These are necessary losses. These losses are celebrated as much as they are mourned. People do experience accidental losses during the first half of life, but generally these are the exceptions to the rule. The vast majority of losses in early life are developmental in nature.

As we enter the second half of life, however, losses take on a different character. The losses that we now experience are more frequent, more permanent, and more negative in nature. They are no longer termed "growth experiences" (although they can be) nor are they always celebrated. Losses also begin to become cumulative in nature after age forty. Losses build upon losses; each loss is linked to previous losses, and in a sense foreshadows the ultimate loss of life itself. We need to understand in particular the losses of the second half of life and how to deal with them in ways that augment our emotional and spiritual health. This is the task of this book.

Before we turn our attention to a discussion of these losses per se, however, we will discuss the nature of grief and the nature of spiritual health. The chapter on grief dynamics is a somewhat brief summary of the nature of grief. For a fuller discussion of this important topic, I refer you to my earlier book, *Grief and Growth: Pastoral Resources for Emotional and Spiritual Growth.*[1] A solid understanding of the nature of grief, along with a perspective on spiritual health, is foundational to our task of forging an "integrated" approach to understanding loss in later life. It is to these subjects that we turn initially, followed by chapters on what I consider to be the key losses of later life. In conclusion, the last chapter will take a wider look at loss and aging from the vantage point of faith.

In this book, I have focused on seven major losses: loss of youth, loss of family, loss of parents, loss of work, loss of spouse, loss of health, and loss of independence. Shorter discussions of several additional losses have been placed in the chapter where they seem best to fit. However, each person's journey is unique. Some readers may find one of these major losses to be relatively minor in their lives. Others may find that a loss to which I have given minor attention has been quite major in their experience. I think, however, that most of us will pass through each of the losses discussed in this book in some form or another.

I would also like to note that I have not placed these losses in any specific chronological order, although some people will argue for such. Each loss is as much a process that colors all of the years of later life as it is a single event. In fact, I would argue that each loss is experienced both as event and as process. That is part of the nature of loss in the later years.

My gratitude goes to the people who have read all or portions of this manuscript and given me helpful feedback. I appreciate your support. I would also like to thank my colleagues and friends at the Walnut Valley Counseling Center, who put up with my absence while I was writing this book. Most important, I am grateful for the many people who have shared their losses with me, as their pastor, friend, and counselor. Many of their stories, appropriately disguised, are included in this book in the hopes that their experiences will enrich all of us. May God bless your reading and your journey.

R. Scott Sullender
Claremont, California

Introduction
to the Second Edition

I was pleasantly surprised by the popularity of the first edition of this book. The book was a successful blend of research and science and personal anecdotes and stories. Its basic pitch is positive: that even though the second half of life is filled with losses, each loss is an opportunity for a deeper spirituality. Or, in other words, every stage of life, even the seemingly worst ones, have the potential for spiritual growth embedded in their very structure. Most of all, the popularity of this book is due to its subject matter. It touches us where we live. We all get older. We all experience various losses, and we all look for ways to keep life enriching, rewarding, and interesting in the midst of it.

I was pleased when Richard Dayringer and The Haworth Press asked me to produce a second edition. Almost from the beginning, I wasn't entirely satisfied with Chapter 9. Thus, in this second edition, I have reworked, retitled, and rewritten this chapter. It is now titled "The Loss of Independence." I am pleased with the result. I believe that it captures well the various aspects of the loss of independence as it is experienced by most people. Besides this change, portions of Chapters 8 and 10 have been rewritten and enhanced, based on new research and the current evolution of my thinking on the subjects.

I hope that all of you who read this book will be enlightened and enriched on your path through the later years of life.

Chapter 1

The Grief Dynamic

... and you will know the truth and the truth will set you free.

Jn 8:32

Grief is, simply put, the human emotion that we feel when we lose someone or something to which we are psychologically attached. It is the feeling of sorrow, sadness, and even nostalgia. It occurs every time there is a loss. Grief is therefore universal among humans. Yet grief feelings can vary widely in intensity, depending on how emotionally attached we were to that which is lost. Obviously, when we lose someone very important to us, we grieve with intensity, very long and very deeply. If, however, we lose something less important to us or something that we have partially accepted as already lost, then our experience of grief is light, subtle, and short-lived. In some of the latter cases we might not notice that we are grieving at all.

GRIEF'S PAIN AND ITS DEFENSES

Grief is painful. That sounds like an obvious statement. Yet, it needs to be emphasized. Grief feelings are painful feelings. The pain may be intense or light, but it is pain. Unlike physical pain, the pain of grief cannot readily be seen nor easily soothed with cold compresses or carefully prescribed medications. Grief is essentially a subjective experience, which is largely in the mind, or shall I say, in the heart of the griever. To the sorrower, the pain of grief is very real and it is as powerful and as influential in his or her life as any physical ailment could be.

Most humans do not like pain and seek to avoid it whenever possible. So too, most of us go to lengths to avoid the pain of grief as well. When we see a loss coming down the road of life, we pretend that it won't happen to us or that it's still too far away to worry about. When we are told that a loss is about to happen, we look for ways to prevent it or to escape its consequences. And when a loss has occurred, we are slow to fully realize that the loss is final, irreversible, and demands adjustments in our lives. It is little wonder then that most people have difficulty with grief. Indeed, it has been my experience that most modern Americans have trouble handling grief feelings. Our efforts to deny it, avoid it, or defer its full impact hamper our ability to be healed in a timely and easy manner.

These mental tricks that we play on ourselves to avoid, deny, or soften the impact of grief's pain, are called by psychologists "defense mechanisms." A defense mechanism is any mental mechanism used by us to shield us from pain, in this case, psychological pain. Defense mechanisms are not all bad. In fact, they are quite necessary. We could not cope with pain without some means of moderating its intensity. Yet a prolonged clinging to defense mechanisms, in the face of a reality that demands the opposite, can lead to serious mental, emotional, and familial problems.

In the context of bereavement, many types of defense mechanisms exist. There are, however, certain common ones.

Denial

Denial is the psychological mechanism whereby we avoid emotionally realizing that the loss has occurred or is about to occur. We deny its reality. We literally pretend it's not there. Denial comes in varying forms and degrees.[1] A first-degree denial, the most serious kind, occurs when a person totally denies the reality of an imminent loss and even denies all of the related facts surrounding its existence. A person who has a terminal illness, for example, may deny that he or she has any illness at all or even has been to the hospital recently. This is the extreme! But the pain of the imminent loss of life is so intense, so devastating that he or she must reject, at least for the moment, all facts related to the situation. It will literally be blotted out.

Another person (or the same person at a later stage of bereavement) may admit cognitively and verbally that the loss has occurred, but emotionally still feels as if it hasn't really happened. This is called a second-degree denial and is characterized by the phrase "It happened, but who cares?" The individual acknowledges the loss, but is emotionally turned off or anesthetized.[2] For example, a grieving wife might say, "I know that he is gone, but I just cannot accept it. It feels as if he's still here, as if he's out there, on a business trip, and will be pulling into the driveway any time now." This type of denial is not as extreme as a first-degree denial and usually leads, in time, to a full realization of the loss. It is as if this woman's emotions need time to catch up with what her mind already knows. Emotions change slower than cognitions.

Third-degree denial occurs when someone (or the same person at a still later stage of bereavement) may admit the reality of the loss cognitively and may even have worked it through emotionally, but still has not fully adjusted to the loss and continues to act as if life is the same as it was prior to the loss. This is the mildest type of denial. People can be slow to make adjustments to their new status or identity. The unemployed man delays seeking a new job. The grieving husband is slow to get rid of his wife's sewing machine or her favorite dresses. The handicapped woman continues to try to do it on her own. Behavior then is the final and slowest part of our lives to accept the full reality of a loss. We can still deny a loss behaviorally long after we have come to accept it, cognitively and emotionally.

Viewed from this perspective, the process of grieving could be understood as passing through different levels of denial.[3] At each stage the griever accepts a little more of the full reality of the loss, until he or she embraces the loss with the whole being. If the loss comes as an unexpected, unwanted tragedy, we may begin with a first-degree denial. We are shocked, numbed by the pain. Gradually, though, we accept the loss cognitively. We know it happened. Then we come to feel it, at first marginally and then deeply. We work it through emotionally. Finally, our behavior catches up with the process and we make the necessary changes that the loss requires. Now we live it.

Generally speaking, denial is a costly defense mechanism. To pretend that something didn't happen, we must distort reality so badly that this distortion itself causes us great psychological harm. In addition, denial requires great psychic energy to maintain, energies that could be spent in productive activity. Second-degree denial, denying our emotions, can also be costly in another sense. It seems to be a truism that if we repress one emotion, we inevitably repress them all. People who cannot or who refuse to grieve are often people who also cannot love. There is little joy, little love, little anger . . . little anything emotionally. They are emotionally dead. Yet, I have found that when these persons start grieving again, they experience a flood of various emotions. Suddenly they are able to feel again—feel anger, feel love, feel joy . . . feel alive.

Rationalization

Rationalization is a defense mechanism whereby we offer explanations for why a loss really isn't so bad. We rationalize the loss so that the pain does not hurt quite so much. We make excuses to and for ourselves. Rationalization is largely a cognitive process. It is a way of comforting ourselves. Rationalizations ease our pain. If we have lost a job, we say, "It really wasn't such a good job after all. The boss was a grouch and the pay was lousy." If we have lost our home, we might say, "I didn't like that neighborhood anyhow. Those teenagers were always so noisy and unruly. We will find a better place to live." If we have lost a parent, we may say, "Well, at least Dad died a peaceful death. He didn't have to suffer on in one of those nursing homes. He wouldn't have wanted that." Each of these statements is designed to alleviate our pain, just a bit, and help us cope with the terrible loss that is now before us.

I do not mean to imply that rationalizations are always false or untrue statements. On the contrary, there is some truth in the previous statements. Looking for the silver lining in tragic events can be a way of empowering and uplifting our spirits. Rationalizations, like all defense mechanisms, are coping devices. Rationalizations distort reality, however slightly, and prevent us from seeing life as it now really is. That may not be all bad, if we need a little fantasy to help us cope for a while. Yet, rationalizations can become walls behind which we hide from our painful feelings. We know that healing lies in facing the pain, in all of its fullness and implications. Healing lies in passing through the pain, not in avoiding it. In time rationalizations should give way to a fuller acceptance of truth and give birth to an affirmation of life amid sorrow.

Idealization

Idealization is a process whereby a grieving person idealizes that which is lost. Here too the griever may distort reality to a degree. In idealization, the griever momentarily forgets the negative attributes of the deceased or the favorite job or whatever he or she has lost and focuses exclusively on what is missed most. Almost all people in grief do some idealizing about the loss. Gradually, however, as the grieving process leads to healing, one remembers a more realistic picture of what was lost.

As an individual who does considerable marriage counseling, I am keenly aware of how many troubled marriages there are in this country. And even among the functional marriages, almost all couples have their points of tension, disagreement, and regret. Yet, when I speak about grief at widows' meetings, I am fascinated by how many wonderful marriages there are in the world. The show of hands or the spontaneous sharing is amazing. Nearly every woman claims in some fashion that her dead husband was the most kind, loyal, and devoted man she knew. Now I ask you, where did all of those troubled marriages go? Surely, the widows of troubled marriages may not be as likely to attend lectures on bereavement as are the widows who had positive marital relationships. It may also be that grief plays tricks on us all. The negative aspects of our marriages or marriage partners fade when the eyes are filled with tears.

Idealization, like other defense mechanisms, can be extreme or very modest in nature.[4] The more extreme idealization is, the more it distorts reality and the more disturbing and damaging it is to our mental health. Idealization, also like other defense mechanisms, is normally more extreme in the early stages of bereavement and gradually gives way, as grieving continues, to the less extreme forms. And in time, if the grief process continues in a positive manner, idealization is replaced by a realistic picture of the loss. The goal of grieving is to accept reality and to see life as it really was with all of the blemishes, all of the beauty, and all of the ambiguities.

Reaction Formation

Reaction formation is a technical, psychoanalytic term for a type of defense mechanism whereby a person has an extreme opposite or displaced reaction to some unacceptable anxiety. I would like to alter the term slightly to include any attempt to run from pain by overemphasizing the opposite i.e., over reaction. Sometimes when we feel the approaching pain of a loss, we run from it. We flee psychologically. Usually this "fleeing" is in an opposite direction from our fear.

Middle-aged persons, for example, may fear losing their jobs, that they are being bypassed by younger colleagues. They respond by becoming more compulsive about their work, workaholics, trying even harder to please the boss in every way. Overactivity can be one way to avoid pain. Again, the key word is "over." Activity is not bad in itself, but only harmful if it prevents us from dealing with our feelings.

Consider the parent who feels anxious about the impending departure of adolescent children. With each passing year, they are getting older, more grown up, more independent. Soon they will be leaving home. The parent responds out of anxiety by clamping down even harder on the teenagers—more rules, more chores, higher expectations, and tighter restrictions. Psychologically, this parent is trying to keep them at home, as children, trying to hold them close just a few more years. Unfortunately, this "controlling" can have the opposite effect. The children may rebel, looking for every opportunity to express their independence or stay away from home. And the more they distance themselves from home, the more anxious the parent becomes, and the tighter the restrictions grow. This cyclic dynamic may escalate to the point of full-scale rebellion and require the intervention of a family therapist. Note that the problem began when the parent sought to avoid painful feelings about an impending loss by fleeing into the opposite. This type of reaction formation is a very common theme among those who grieve.

Substance Abuse

People can also flee or run away psychologically in countless other ways. Regression refers to a way of fleeing pain by going backward to a younger state of mind or way of behaving. Drug and alcohol abuse has regressive themes to it, particularly when it is used to cope with loss experiences. Alcohol is a common way of deadening pain, calming fears, and making reality go away. Alcohol is one way to anesthetize pain. It is no accident that most people's consumption of alcohol goes up during bereavement. The pain is gone temporarily. The next day, of course, the pain is there again. Pain never goes away permanently through any defense mechanism. Pain does not go away if you run away, but sometimes we need to anesthetize pain for a while (we are buying some time), while we build up our courage to face reality. If any defense mechanism becomes permanent, then we have only encased pain, not eliminated it. We have ceased to grow, because we have failed to grieve. This is one of the main ways that people become psychologically and spiritually crippled.

I hope that it is clear from this brief description of defense mechanisms and other assorted coping devices that grief feelings are painful feelings and that one way to understand the different approaches people have to grief is to view their behavior as ways of coping with pain. This will be an important observation to keep in mind as we approach a discussion of loss and grief in later life. By the time we have reached the second half of life, most of us have some pretty well-established ways of coping with emotional pain. Some of these coping mechanisms may be healthy; others may not be so helpful. In general, the pain needs to be dealt with emotionally if we wish to be healed. Each person, however, will find a different approach and pace to that process. Most successful grieving is a gentle combination of "facing the pain" and "distancing from the pain," a process that gradually moves toward restoration.

THE PROCESS OF GRIEVING

It shoul be clear by now is that grief is a process. This is a fairly simple, but important concept. Grief does not stay the same from day to day or week to week. It moves. It changes. It is like a journey down a winding road, wherein each turn in the path reveals a new landscape . . . or a landscape that you thought you left three stages ago.[5] The critical issue is to keep moving down the path. The temptation is always to retreat to a safe spot. Yet healing comes only as we continue down that pathway, "through the valley of the shadow of death," and we move through this valley only by regularly processing our feelings.

What makes this grieving journey even more interesting and complex is the mixture of other emotions that get added into the process.

Grief itself, pure and simple, is the sensation of longing, sorrowing, and yearning. Yet, the *grief process* is a collection of feelings and emotions, of which grief is the most dominant, but not the only emotion. The following are some of the more common emotional companions.

Anger is a familiar element in bereavement, especially when the loss is unwanted. We protest. We argue. We get mad at everyone and everything. We look for someone to blame. We feel angry that our loved one was taken from us, or that we cannot work anymore, or that our children do not call us as often as we would like or that our bodies do not work the way they used to. Anger is a normal feeling in bereavement, but difficult for many people to acknowledge and allow themselves to express.

Depression is also a fellow traveler with us along the road of sorrow. Depression comes on us because we hold in some of that anger. We internalize it instead of expressing it. We may feel angry with ourselves or at the deceased or at God—all of whom are uncomfortable objects to be angry at. Periods of depression are common in bereavement, but they usually lift as the feelings are expressed and processed.

Despair is a close cousin to depression, but is more future oriented than depression. There are times in bereavement when we feel hopeless about life. Our future now looks bleak, limited, and dark. We have lost the one thing or one person we loved most. Despair, particularly in old age, is much more difficult to cure than depression. Ultimately the only cure is the one that comes when we pass into a new stage of life and embrace life again as "good." Unfortunately, many people in later life, as I will suggest, do not make those many transitions and gradually sink into a chronic state of despair.

Guilt is another inevitable emotion in sorrow, particularly certain types of losses. Humans want to know why something tragic happened. "Why" questions reflect our desire to understand our personal responsibility in the events that have transpired. We ask, "What did I do wrong that caused this loss?" or "Did I say something I should not have?" or "Did I make the right decisions?" or the perpetual "What if" question: "What if I had done this or said that?" "What if I had worked harder or driven safer or raised them differently? Could this loss have been avoided?" Those are all typical and inevitable questions. The situations vary, but the need to ask the questions remains.

One of the ongoing themes of grief work in later life is untangling the confusion people feel over their relative responsibility for past losses.

Anxiety and its more specific cousin, fear, are also present in grief. Anxiety comes to us first as a loss approaches. We anticipate losses, and as we do so, we get anxious. We do not wish to lose what we value. We do not want to be hurt. As I see my body change, I get anxious. As I watch my children grow up, I feel anxious. As I see younger colleagues flourish, I feel anxious. All of these signs of approaching loss cause anxiety.

A type of fear or anxiety that is present in bereavement is post-loss. As we move through bereavement, we begin to worry about the unknown future that now lies before us because we have lost a loved one. We do not know what will happen to us now. "How will I cope now without her?" "How will I find enough money to live on in retirement?" "How will I get along with a crippled body?" "Will my children still love me after they leave?" These are the questions, prompted by fear, that linger in bereavement. Fears of loneliness, dependency, financial insecurity, and declining health increase with every loss in the later years.

All of these emotions, along with grief itself, can be present in the grief process. The most critical factor in the resolution of these emotions, including grief, is the full expression of these feelings. The verbalization of feelings is the God-given way we have to process our emotions. It is also the typically and uniquely human way. Generally speaking, the more we verbalize the better. The more we talk about or express these feelings, the more our grief process will move along toward some resolution. The temptation is to hold it in, to be silently strong, to not want to bother anyone with our troubles, to run away from the painful sorrow or the angry reactions or the nagging guilt. Such temptations hamper our healing. As Jesus suggests in the second beatitude, only as we mourn will we find comfort (Mt 5:4). It is better to allow ourselves to grieve, as fully and as completely as possible. Grief is much like a river that flows by itself toward the goal of restoration. Trying to block the river is difficult and ultimately self-destructive, but stepping into the river, flowing with the current, will move us along toward healing. In fact, generally speaking, the more we grieve, the easier and quicker we will come out of it. It is a strange but true paradox.

GRIEF AND MEANING

Grief is a function of attachment. Humans have an innate "instinct" to emotionally attach ourselves to various people, objects, things, places. We care. That is part of the nature of being human.[6] Whenever we invest ourselves in something or someone, we infuse it with meaning. We say that we find it meaningful. We value it. We build our lives, our identities, our values around such "attachments." So, when we lose those attachments, for whatever reason, we must to some extent restructure our meanings, our values, even our identities. Grieving therefore can be understood as having a spiritual or theological dimension to it. That dimension can best be described as a process of giving up, readjusting, and/or finding new meaning in one's life.

One of the least studied and least understood areas of human psychology has to do with meaning. Humans, unlike other animals, have a "will to meaning."[7] We need to have a sense of meaning and purpose to be psychologically sound. "Meaning" is a difficult term to define. Generally, meaning refers to a set of beliefs, what I call operational beliefs, that place the individual's life within a larger context. The realm of meaning, when it is functioning well, provides the individual with: (a) a sense of purpose, (b) a sense of personal significance, (c) a set of values and corresponding rationales, (d) a sense of identity. Meaning is largely a cognitive function. Meaning is made up of beliefs or cognitions. Yet as noted above, meaning also has an emotional dimension. Things that we become emotionally attached to, we term "meaningful," and we surround those attachments with certain beliefs that explain their importance to us. Attachment, then, is a way of talking about meaning, at least the emotional part of one's meaning system.

Traditionally, meanings has been provided for us by our religion, our culture, and/or other institutions. Some people find great meaning, for example, in their family. Others find meaning in their work. Others find it in their religious beliefs, and still others, in an avocation or cherished cause. Some find their greatest meaning to be in their appearance or financial status. Meaning is largely a subjective phenomenon. Individuals can get a sense of meaning in their lives from an infinite variety of sources, but the need for meaning is universal.

In the twentieth-century Westernized cultures, most of the traditional sources of meaning—religion, nation, work, and family—are changing rapidly and losing their ability to communicate values and command allegiance. Many of the traditional beliefs and symbols are no longer relevant to many people. In an increasingly pluralistic culture the problem is complicated even further. As a result, more and more modern, particularly urban, people are experiencing an existential emptiness or meaninglessness. It is a frightening thing to realize that one's life is essentially without value, that one's life is really insignificant, and that all of one's life work counts for naught. More and more people seem to feel this way, and seem to be on a search for a more lasting sense of purpose.

When we lose something of significance, we are thrown into what I call a "crisis of meaning." We are temporarily without a sense of purpose. Our life may seem unimportant. Grief sufferers may say, "My life has no value, now that Susie is gone." Or, "I feel so worthless now that I am not a contributing member of society." Or "It feels pointless to keep on living now that I can't care for myself. I'm only a burden to my family."

Most of us find our self-worth in life from several sources simultaneously. We have families, careers, hobbies, religious beliefs, political activities, etc. If we lose one of these areas, we have other areas to fall back on. But what about the man who has "put all of his eggs in one basket," for example, investing all of his energy into his career? Will it not be more difficult for him to adjust to retirement than for other men? Or what of the woman who has overinvested herself in her family and parenting? Will it not be more difficult for her to adjust to the "empty nest" than for the woman who has also invested herself in a career or in some political/social cause? Or consider the man who has overinvested himself in his appearance. To him looking healthy, trim, and handsome is everything! It will be much more difficult for him to deal with his loss of youth than for the man who also invested himself in a career, in his education, and/or in family relations. My point is that losses create mini spiritual crises, and if what we have lost is central to our value system, then our crisis will be great. The meaning factor is an important element in understanding a person's grief reaction.

By the time most of us have reached age forty, we have some well-established value systems, which are usually focused around the major areas of life—family, work, health, friends. Most of us know who we are, what we value, and from where we derive our sense of purpose. But during the second half of life, we will suffer losses in each one of these major areas; family, work, marriage, health, status, friends, etc. Inevitably then, these losses will lead us to reevaluate, rethink, or redo our value systems. Each loss in later life carries with it this kind of spiritual or theological "crisis." We will ask questions such as, "What is the meaning of this loss?" and "What does my life mean now that I am without what I've lost?" and "Can life be good again?" These questions reflect the spiritual "limbo" that most people feel themselves to be in while grieving. Finding answers to these questions is an important part of the healing process.

GRIEF IN LATER LIFE

Grief does seem to become more complex, more intense, and more chronic in later life. There are some unique themes to loss and grief in the later years. As we enter those years ourselves or work with people going through those stages of life, we need to understand the uniqueness of grief in the later years. Here are some themes.

Rapidity of Losses

Losses come faster in later life. For example, consider the loss of a friend or relative by death. Although distant relatives die with some regularity, the death of a peer is usually rare in early life. Yet after the passage of the midlife point, we begin to notice that more of our peers die of heart attacks, cancer, or other natural causes. These events are no longer rare or accidental. And in old age, the death of peers becomes a regular occurrence. The longer we live, the more we experience the death of friends, peers, and colleagues.

Consider also health-related losses. Young people rarely experience a permanent loss of health. But as we grow old, we begin to notice minor physical limitations and annoyances. Still later, we experience the first semipermanent or permanent loss of health. Perhaps we now need eyeglasses. Perhaps our digestive tract needs regular assistance. Perhaps our muscles need massage, or the right ear needs a hearing aid. Each of these losses demands an adjustment from us. We barely have adjusted to the last loss before a new one is upon us.

Losses seem to increase geometrically the longer we live. This makes the grieving process that much more complicated. Most people grieve slowly and incompletely, in spite of the best psychological advice to the contrary. That is OK when there is only one loss a year, but what happens when there are three losses a year? Now the grieving process backs up.

Roger was still adjusting to his mother's death when he was forced to take an early retirement for health reasons. Now he has three major losses he is dealing with, all within a short four-year period. He used to say to me in the midst of all this, "One of these losses would have been enough for a guy like me. I really don't do very well with emotional stuff. Now I feel as though I have more than I can cope with." Roger was not coping well and the increased rapidity of losses in later life was catching up with him. He had to learn new, more rapid ways of dealing with loss.

Losses come upon losses in later life—one grief, and then another. Some people, such as Roger, just cannot keep up with it. It overwhelms their limited processing skills. Those who do learn to stay mentally healthy in later life do so because they learn, or have learned, to grieve well and grieve rapidly.

Finality of Losses

Losses are more final in the later years. If we lose our spouse early in our life, there is still time to remarry and resume a normal life. Yet, if we lose our spouse in the later years, there is less chance of remarriage. Women, for example, who lose their husband by divorce or by death after age fifty, seldom remarry.[8] This is a fact that crosses the minds of many troubled couples who contemplate divorce after midlife. Similarly, if a man loses his job in the early years of his life, it is a momentary hardship at worst. But if a man who is fifty-seven years old or older loses his job, there is little time left to find a new career. Many men in this age bracket, who work for large competitive companies, are afraid to request even a small job change lest they give their employer the excuse to let them go. "Who is going to want an individual with barely ten years of active employment left?" they reason. Their reasoning isn't all that unrealistic in many competitive markets.

Losses in later life have this sense of finality that the losses in earlier life did not have. In fact, this finality permeates all of the losses of later life, even the relatively minor ones.

The Ever-Present Character of Loss

Loss is more subtle and everpresent in later life. Loss is with us all the time of course, but in later life it seems as though there are fewer big dramatic losses and more of the gradual, subtle, constant losses. Most of the losses of later life are anticipated or should be. We know that someday our health will fail. Someday our spouse will pass on. Someday we will retire. There are often long periods of anticipation before these losses actually occur. This can be a very positive occurrence. It gives us time to prepare, if we will. But because the losses are more subtle, more diffuse, they are also easier to ignore for the person bent on avoidance. We can put off thinking about retirement or about what we are going to do when Mother dies or where will we live when Sarah's eyes go. These are painful questions, easy questions to put off until tomorrow.

Because of these losses, grief is everpresent. Older people are almost in a constant state of grief. There is always a loss or two that they are adjusting to and always a loss or two just over the horizon that they are anticipating. Grief is a constant companion in the later years. The well-adjusted person in later life will learn to make friends with grief. In fact, I would argue that if we want to age well through the second half of life we must become good grievers. We must learn to work through our ever-present grief.

Losses Are Cumulative

Losses become more cumulative in the later years. It is not uncommon to attend a funeral in later life and find oneself crying, not over the current loss, but over an old one. The present grieving triggers past grieving in us. Current memories help us remember past hurts. Emotionally, losses seem to be linked together, like a long chain-link fence. Pull at one post and all of the posts vibrate.

This cumulative nature of loss and grief makes grieving more difficult in later life. We are not just grieving one loss, but several losses. With each passing year, many older adults leave more and more losses ungrieved. Some losses can never be fully and completely resolved. What this does mean, however, is that most of us have grief feelings just below the surface of our psyches. Unconsciously, we know this and therefore seek to avoid further losses or grief rites all the more. We fear that we could easily become overwhelmed by all of the hurt within us. This is the cumulative nature of losses in later life.

LOSS IS SUBJECTIVE

Loss is largely a subjective experience. Two people may experience the same event, but one person labels it a "loss" and the other person labels it a "transition." Every loss, even the most tragic, has some positive elements. Most losses actually carry with them a mixture of feelings—negative feelings of grief, sorrow, guilt, and fear, and the positive feelings of relief, and anticipation of freedom.

In addition, individuality increases with age. We are not all the same, and in fact we become more unique, the older we get. What this means is that the variety of ways people approach and experience loss also increases with age. Some people will look upon retirement as a loss; many others will see it as a blessing and still others as simply a transition. The empty-nest stage may be experienced by some adults as a negative event and by others as a new sense of personal freedom. Some will mourn. Others will rejoice. Most will feel elements of both. What this also means is that no one's advice about losses in later life, especially mine, will apply uniformly to everyone. Everyone's experience is slightly different. I believe, however, that everyone's experience of loss in later life will involve some elements of grief. The grief may be more keenly felt at certain times than others. Inevitably it will be there, and unless or until it is dealt with, we cannot pass on into the next stage of life.

Perhaps "loss" is not the best word at all to describe the events of this book. Perhaps "transition" or "change" better characterize the flavor of these events. Every loss is, after all, a change and a transition. Every loss carries with it "a demand," a requirement that we must change. But before we can change, we must first grieve the loss. Before we can go forward, we must go backward. Grieving comes first. Grieving makes growing possible.

Chapter 2

Spiritual Health and Grief

For where your treasure is, there will be your heart also.

Mt 6:21

What does the model Christian look like? How would you describe the ideal religious person? In response to such questions, people of faith will paint widely differing pictures. There are probably as many different descriptions of this imaginary person as there are denominations or religious traditions. Each group, and maybe even each individual, will have an unique vision of the goal toward which we strive as pilgrims along the Way. The other interesting and related question is, "Does spiritual health change with the differing stages of life? Are the qualities that make one spiritually mature the same for the sixteen-year-old as they are for the forty-eight-year-old?" The question is certainly an intriguing one.

In this book I am going to propose a definition of spiritual health based on the concept of idolatry. Idolatry is a theme throughout the Scriptures and, in slightly differing forms, throughout the history of Christianity. It is a doctrine that challenges our basic understanding of God and human nature. It is a concept that both Jews and Christians can ascribe to as central to their understanding of God. Most important, it is a definition of spiritual health that can transcend the differing stages of the life cycle. In this chapter I will describe the basics of our theological understanding of idolatry, indicating how this view of spiritual health might enrich our understanding of grief and loss in the later years.

MAKING GODS

Idolatry is simply the "worshiping of false gods." It appears in the Ten Commandments, in the fiery sermons of Ezekiel, in the Maccabean revolt, in Jesus' teachings against Pharisaic legalisms, and there in Paul's advice to Gentile Christians. All of Scripture could be understood as God's struggle with humans over idolatry. Humans seem to fashion idols for themselves over and over again. Each time the false gods get the upper hand, God breaks through our idolatry, calling us to a renewed faith in God alone. These brief periods of freedom, however, seem to be only interludes before we again fashion some new kind of idol.

In the period of the Old Testament, people fashioned images from clay or stone, which they then worshipped. Idol is derived from the Greek word *eidōlon,* which means "image." These statues were concrete visualizations of the imagined gods, be they the wind or rain or the gods of Canaan or the gods of fertility or prosperity. There were usually many gods, each having its own "turf" or area of authority. In a sense the battle between faith and idolatry, especially during Israel's years as a nation, was a battle between monotheism and polytheism. There were periods when both theological systems co-existed. People believed that "the Lord God is one," but they also visited local shrines and paid homage to lesser gods. Idolatry was also a nationalistic issue in ancient Israel. Monotheism was Israel's religion, whereas the religions of Israel's neighbors were polytheistic. The plea to return to a faith in one God often had nationalistic overtones. Abhorrence of idols and idolatry runs deep within the veins of Judaism and Jews.

In the Gospels we find few clay statues, but idolatry is just as critical an issue. Now idolatry takes the more subtle, but equally powerful forms of legalism, greed, lust, and false allegiances. When Jesus confronts the rich young ruler (Lk 18:18-30), he is challenging him to give up his worship of wealth. When Jesus preaches to the scribes and Pharisees, he calls them to replace the god of legalism with a true faith in God that transcends the law. People may not be publicly "bowing down" before idols, but they still are creating and worshipping false gods in their hearts. They may attend formal worship services for the one God, but their informal, daily allegiances are elsewhere. Again, we find idolatry and faith existing side by side and the struggle between the two continuing into the Christian era. Now, the battleground is no longer the institutional structures of religion and state, but the hearts, lives, and souls of individual persons. The issue is no longer the concrete idols, but the human tendency to create and worship false gods.

Biblical history can be characterized as a constant struggle between idolatry and faith, between worshiping the false gods and worshiping "the living God." The form of the struggle changes slightly with each generation, but the struggle continues.

Let me raise the questions then, Why is there such a struggle at all? Why don't humans learn their lesson once and for all? Humans don't learn because something about human nature drives us to "make gods." Repeatedly, humans create false gods to worship. Even when we have formally pledged our allegiance to the living God, we still can't stop ourselves from this tendency to create and cling to false gods. I would suggest, as do the Scriptures, that humans "need" false gods. Idol making is fueled by our innate insecurity with human existence itself, with our creatureliness, with our perceived powerlessness over the forces that control us. Fueled by this anxiety, we are driven "to idolize."

Anything, even good things, can be made into a god, especially in the context of bereavement. I was asked once by the conference minister to intercede as a meditator in a dispute between two segments of a local church. These kinds of "church wars" are always difficult to deal with. The two segments of the congregation were divided sharply regarding the issue of pastoral leadership. One group was extremely loyal to the former minister who had served that congregation for eighteen years, had retired the previous year, and then died unexpectedly two months later. The other group was supportive of the new cleric, who was struggling to find his own identity amid a congregation that was dominated by the ghost of the former minister. Other issues were operating here as well. The former group was largely older; the latter group, younger. The former group consisted of long-term members; the latter group were mostly newer members. And there were some individual grudges thrown into the controversy as well. All in all it was quite a war; it split the congregation right down the middle.

This conflict was triggered by a request rename the church after the former pastor. To the older members it was a wonderful suggestion, a noble tribute to a man who had given so much of his life serving these people. The current pastor, supported by the other segment of the congregation, discouraged the idea. To him it seemed a bit too much, "rather as though we are glorifying the dead or something." His remarks were met with anger and hurt by the former group, who could easily recount story upon story of the wonders of their former pastor. The current pastor was reluctant to "put his foot down." He didn't want to lose this older, more influential segment of the congregation— but neither did he want the church renamed after his predecessor.

These situations are not easily resolved, and this one was particularly difficult. A compromise was found eventually that saved the church's unity, but not without the price of a few members. However, I remember being impressed with how easily believers can idolize ("make little gods of") people, even good ones. In this case the process was fueled by the pain of grief and idealization of the deceased. Release and wholeness came only when God broke through to several mourning members, with a vision of faith in Christ that transcends loyalty to persons.

Religious people are not immune from this tendency to create and worship false gods. Even though we formally worship the living God, we can nevertheless create one or many "little gods" that in fact may have more influence in our lives than the true God. The Christian walk is a constant struggle to stay on the "straight and narrow path" and avoid the many temptations to worship elsewhere.

TEMPORARY GODS

Idolatry occurs when something that is less than God is set up as a god. Nearly anything can be made into a god. In ancient times it was the attributes of nature—there were sun gods and gods of thunder and gods that dwelt in the ocean depths. Political entities could also be made into gods. Caesar was treated like a god, as were the pharaohs of Egypt. Desired qualities can become gods. There were fertility gods that bestowed children and/or a good harvest on their devoted subjects. Beauty might be made into a little god and would hopefully grant lovliness to its faithful. In more modern times, we find people who worship success, fame, power, status, and wealth. They live for their gods just as surely as the ancients did for theirs.

Whether ancient or modern, however, idols are always essentially temporary, not eternal. Rulers die. Fame fades. Success is short-lived. And fertility is only for a season. Idols are false gods precisely because they are finite. They are of this world. Yet by making these things into gods, we hope they will become infinite. Of course, they never do. They are relative, not absolute; temporary, not permanent.

Marlene sat in my office sobbing. She was a broken woman, a desperate woman. She cried out, "Nobody! Nobody will take me seriously, doctor. I am more than a cute face and a big set of boobs. I have a brain! I have an intellect. I have a soul!" Yes, that is what Marlene needed, to claim her lost soul. As she poured out her history, she told me that from day one in her life, she was told how cute she was. She was the apple of her parents' eye, the youngest and prettiest of six children. She was fussed over. She was dressed up. She was admired. She was entered in all of the beauty contests and usually won. Always she was expected just to stand there and look pretty. Don't say anything. Don't do anything. Just look good. And so she did. As she grew into adulthood, she incorporated those values. She too worshiped at the altar of appearance. She spent hours in front of the mirror, among the clothes' racks, and in the beauty salons.

The only trouble with this scheme was that Marlene grew older, and at thirty-eight her beauty was dull compared to the sparkling looks of younger women. She began to have a growing sense of emptiness, at times even of panic. Part of her wanted it back—the attention, the youth, the admiration. Part of her was angry—angry that she was deluded, angry that she couldn't stay young no matter how hard she tried, angry that she had nothing else going for her. The cruelty was that she both hated it and loved it. Her beauty was her blessing and her curse.

It was hard for Marlene to break free from the grip of this false god, particularly in a society that worships at the same altar. Her liberation however begun when she started to see that the god was temporary, not permanent. Freedom emerged when she began to see that the god's power was waning. Then, and only then, did she begin to reclaim her power.

The fact that false gods are essentially temporary in nature, in contrast to the living God who is eternal, is a helpful distinction to keep in mind as we approach a discussion of loss in later life. We grieve over "attachments" in life that are temporary. We know that someday our health will decline, our job will be terminated, our children will grow up, and our parents will pass on before us. That doesn't stop us, nor should it stop us, from continuing to love such things. But when these attachments are taken from us, it should help us resist the temptation to make them into "little gods."

GODS YOU CAN TOUCH

Another central feature of idolatry is that these lesser gods are almost always concrete or visible entities. They are things of this world that can be directly touched, seen, or grasped. The carved stone idol can be touched. The fury of the ocean can be seen. The armies of imperial Rome can be grasped. False gods are false precisely because they are visible, concrete things of this world. You may recall Isaiah's satire against idolatry in which he describes how the idol maker fashions the idol out of wood and metal and then "falls down to it and worships it and prays to it, 'Deliver me, for thou art my god.'" (Is 44). Isaiah correctly notes that idols are always concrete entities. That is their falsity, but it is also their lure. Their concreteness makes it possible for humans to relate to these gods. They can be captured, held, possessed, even owned.

Idols, the visible representation of false gods, are concrete, but, more than this, the rewards of worshiping false gods are also concrete. If we worship the god of power, we hope to gain the tangible benefits of status, money, and control over our future. If we worship the god of a particular social cause, we hope to see results of that movement's progress in the real world. And if we worship the subtle god, called "being a good boy or girl," we expect to reap the rewards of staying out of trouble and avoiding conflict. It is little wonder then that idols have their appeal. Their rewards are much more real, tangible, and useful than those of an invisible God.

The concrete nature of false gods stands in contrast to the living God, who is essentially invisible. "God is fundamentally, essentially invisible," writes Jacques Ellul.[1] "Over and over again it is proclaimed and stated that no one can see God and live." Even Moses sees God only from behind, as God passes by. No one can see God's face. Normally, we "see only God's trace after he has passed by: God's work and God's action after the fact."[2] Worshiping this kind of God requires great trust. It is much easier for humans to worship the false gods, who are more concrete and whose benefits are more tangible.

Among all of the most popular false gods today, none is more real, down to earth, than money. Bill was particularly prone to the idolization of money. He was raised in a poor home and "had to do without" over and over again. He came to resent being poor and vowed that he would never be such again. After a brief period at college, he left college for the real world of stock trading. He enjoyed the challenge of achievement and the chance to make a fortune. He began by cleaning rooms at night. He studied hard. He asked questions. He learned the business and advanced regularly. When I met Bill he was approaching midlife and "just about had it made." He had a personal portfolio that was going to enable him to retire comfortably at age fifty, if he just made one or two more big trades.

The temptation was just too great. He began to do what every stock trader does at some time or another. He began to cut corners—register stocks at different prices than they were actually sold for. A common practice? "Everyone does it," he thought. He got caught and was fired from his job after twenty-three years in the business. He was shattered. He was depressed, but he couldn't let go. He couldn't walk away; the fear of being poor was too great. It drove him to run the risk again, take that last chance. When I last heard from Bill, he had obtained another job in the same line of work and was moving up the ladder again, still gripped by the vision of "never being poor again." He couldn't see that there was anything else to life, anything else that was so concrete. I wondered when the next crisis would occur.

Jacques Ellul's book *Humiliation of the Word* has offered us a provocative discussion of idolatry in the context of modern technological society. Ellul has argued that God is essentially a God of the word and that idolatry always involves a substituting of something visible for something heard. Modern technological societies are increasingly "humiliating" the spoken word in favor of the visible image, says Ellul. Humans seem to find the visible image easier to relate to, to grasp, and to manipulate. The God of Israel, however, is essentially invisible and therefore unable to be manipulated. Worshiping this God requires more trust, even more faith, than worshiping the visible gods of this world.

FALSE PROMISES

All gods promise salvation. That is part of the definition of god-hood. Gods are sources of salvation. God or gods save us from something dreadful, something we cannot save ourselves from. False gods or idols also promise salvation. That's their lure. The false god always says in so many words, "If you worship me, I will give you all this . . ." The "goodies" may include protection, as from accidents or illnesses or nature's fury. The goodies may be rewards, as a greater harvest or prosperity or a long life. The goodies also may be transcendence or fame or power or "the good life."

The false god's appeal is always to something we need or feel we need to survive. Most of these needs, in proper perspective, are normal human needs. We need food, safety, self-esteem, love, and a sense of transcendence. The idol's lure is that one or more of these needs will be ultimately satisfied once and for all. We need no longer live "by daily bread." Now, we can have it all and have it forever. Finally, we will be genuinely happy. Salvation is just around the corner, if . . .

Television commercials are an interesting commentary on our society. They reflect and sometimes create the needs and the idols of our culture. It is enlightening to examine the promises that television commercials make and the hidden god that they invite us to worship. Consider the following examples:

The beer commercial that shows happy people, having fun, partying together. What does it promise? It promises friendship, if we drink their beer. Is that where friendship is found? What is the god? The god is consumption, alcohol, or pleasure.

The new car commercial shows a person (happy, of course) speeding around curves and over highways and byways. What is the lure? Power, a sense of mastery over the environment, and in a sense over ourselves. What is the hidden god? Control? Worship that god of control and be in command of your life!

The Christmas toy commercials show children opening gifts, responding to the generous parent with kisses and praise. Here the promise is that your children will love you if you buy them these toys. Can love be purchased? Some god would want us to believe so.

A shaving cream commercial shows a man shaving his beard without pain and a sexy woman admiring his smooth skin. What does this product promise? Not just a clean shave, but sex appeal. If you smell right, look right, feel right, you will be desirable. What is the god that they invite you to worship? Sexual satisfaction? Popularity?

Most of us who have been born after 1950 have been raised on television commercials. Researchers say that by the time we are eighteen years old, we have watched 17,000 hours of commercials.[3] That is a lot of brainwashing. These false gods have wonderful marketing programs. The promises seem so inviting, if only they were true.

It would be naive for us to say that false gods do not exist. They exist psychologically. In that sense they control. They influence. They exercise power over individuals. They even enslave, psychologically. They do all of this because they are able to offer a kind of present-day salvation.

They exist—and yet they don't exist—in any broader, or theological framework. This is what Ellul calls the "paradox of idols." They are human creations, products of our own anxieties, and therefore, temporary, limited, finite, and concrete. Their promises are short-sighted.

A CADRE OF SLAVES

All of us have our little obsessions to a certain degree. Most reasonable people can resist the temptation to get too caught up in the worship of false gods. Others cannot. Did you ever look closely at people caught in the trap of idolatry? Such people are compulsive. They are intense, serious, driven to make their sacrifice. Little humor or frivolity is found in their lives, especially about their "ultimate concern."

In a psychological sense these people are slaves. Instead of freeing humans, these gods seem to entrap us. They make us slaves. Clinically this happens because false gods essentially fail to produce the promised salvation, but they do give us just enough to keep us "hooked."[4] If you are an ancient person, who is worshiping the river god and faithfully tossing your sacrifice upon the river once a month, the river responds positively often enough (pure probability) encouraging you to continue. If the river does not respond or floods your farm, then you conclude: "I must have done something wrong. I'll try a bigger sacrifice next month." If you are a modern person who is worshiping the god of perfectionism, you can be perfect just often enough to be pleasing—but never perfect enough. And if you cannot be perfect, well then, "It must be because I didn't try hard enough, or didn't organize my time well enough. Next time I'll be perfect."

People who worship false gods are driven. They are desperate, addicted, narrowly focused. The false god becomes their whole life. It consumes all of their energies. All other values and priorities fade in comparison.

Karen was a perfectionist. She was a nurse by trade, and a good nurse at that. She was head nurse of a demanding section of a major metropolitan hospital. Her perfectionism worked well at the hospital, where everything could be neatly organized, the rounds could be efficiently scheduled, and each job thoroughly completed. The doctors and hospital administrators, who were minor perfectionists themselves, heaped praise upon Karen for her work.

Fortunately (or unfortunately) Karen's religion fed into this drive for perfection. She was a lifelong, active member of a conservative, moralistic church that had extensive instructions on how to live a Christian life. It taught her doctrines of proper beliefs, healthy foods, financial planning, sexual morals, family devotions, and so on. There weren't too many areas of Karen's life that weren't controlled or guided by her church. All that suited her fine. She enjoyed the sense of satisfaction in seeing a job done well and righteously. Her life was well ordered, disciplined, and above reproach.

The only area of Karen's life that wasn't working for her was her home life. Karen's perfectionism drove her husband crazy. He was by nature a much more casual, relational, and even disorganized person. In the early years of their marriage, it really didn't bother him if she wanted to be superwoman. As the children grew and discipline became an issue, however, their two parenting styles clashed head-on. Karen wanted the children's lives well organized and managed for success. Bob was more concerned that the children enjoy themselves. "After all," he would say, "they are only kids once."

With the passing of each year, Karen's need for perfection at home seemed to increase. She became more and more demanding, nagging, and pushing. In return, Bob became more passive aggressive in personality, saying, "Sure, sure, honey. . . ." but then doing nothing. This only aggravated Karen and made her push harder, to which Bob responded by slowing down even more. The children were caught in the middle and soon learned to play one parent against the other.

Merle R. Jordan has suggested in his book that pastoral counseling can be defined as a process of "taking on the gods."[5] People who are disturbed are such because they have given allegiance to some false god that falsely defines who they are and distorts their values and relationships. All of us, says Jordan, have an operational theology that may stand in contrast to our formal or professed theology. Our operational theology includes the beliefs that we actually use to operate our lives. Karen operated her life by the belief that "I am not a worthwhile person unless I am perfect." Unfortunately she could never be completely perfect. So the terror of being worthless drove her . . . and drove her. She never got better until she stopped, turned around, looked the terror in the face, and challenged her basic operational belief about her worthlessness. In short, she never got better until she was willing to "take on the gods."

GOD SEEKS AFTER US

The true living God hates idolatry. God is exclusive, even jealous. This is the message that Scripture gives us over and over again. Idolatry angers God. God created humans to be free, not slaves. God created humans for living relationships, not sterile robotic relationships with cold pieces of stone. God also is angry that some of His children prefer slavery to freedom.[6] God made us free, free to choose slavery over freedom . . . yes, free even to be slaves. According to the Bible, God has not given up on us. God works actively to lure humans away from the worship of false gods. Sometimes that luring is gentle and gradual. Sometimes it is dramatic and traumatic.

Johnny drank alcohol most of his life, as did his brother and his father. Johnny could recount story after story of what fun he had drinking at college parties. In those days, it never occurred to him that this was a problem. Initially, his wife drank as well. That's what he liked about her. However, after the children came, she "got religion" and sobered up, but all of her efforts to get Johnny to sober up failed. After all, Johnny "never took orders from any female," and he "could stop any time he really wanted to."

Johnny's addiction was a special kind of slavery. It was more than a psychological and spiritual addiction, although it was that too. After years of drinking, Johnny was also addicted physically to booze. The "demon" had a special grip on his body as well as on his psyche and soul.

Many people tried subtle ways to lure Johnny away from booze. His pastor spoke to him. His doctor warned him. His wife nagged him. His business partners advised him. None of this worked. Finally, his seven-year-old daughter, lying in her hospital room, got to him when she said, "Daddy, will you stop drinking? You are hurting me." That did it! That and the fact that he had almost killed her in a car accident because he wasn't clear headed enough to react to the other car that was running a red light. The driver of that car, ironically, was booked for drunk driving. Now, Johnny has stopped drinking. With the help of an AA program, he knows that he can never drink again. And if that wasn't enough, he has only to look at the scar on his daughter's arm to remind himself again.

God doesn't intend that anyone, especially a seven-year-old child, be injured or crippled. Then again, idolatry carries with it its own judgment. Sometimes that judgment is harsh. For Johnny, looking at it now from the vantage point of years of sobriety, it was a measure of grace, not judgment. Now Johnny believes that nothing else would have broken him of his fierce addiction to alcohol. "God never gave up on me," says Johnny. "He kept after me. And when gentle ways did not work, God had to be rough with me . . . nothing else would have done it." God is persistent about those He loves.

IDOLATRY AND ABNORMAL GRIEF

As has been noted in Chapter 1, every loss, no matter how major or minor, forces us to enter a grieving process. We mourn for what we have lost. Most people recover well enough. Others do not. Perhaps you have met a few people who remain in grief beyond a reasonable period of time. Such people still cling to the past, longing for the return of the deceased spouse, the lost career, the youthful appearance, the physical potency, in short, "the good old days." Locked in by their sorrow, trapped, even enslaved,[7] these people believe that the only happiness they have ever known or will know is now lost. The future looks bleak. They would rather live in the past.

Clinically, abnormal grief has all of the characteristics of idolatry. If we cannot successfully grieve the loss of something or someone, we may make it into an idol. We may idealize it beyond all semblances to what it really was. We "idolize" it. We long for it. We want it back. We believe that it alone will give us happiness, only if it returns . . . or only if we continue to give it our allegiance. We can't let go. The more intense our fixation becomes, the more we are driven by it. We may become consumed by the loss. Nothing else matters. Our priorities, our values, are altered to accommodate this obsession with the past. It has become our false god.

People who are stuck in abnormal grief fail to see that they have "idolized" their loss. The lost person or entity, no matter how dear it is to them, has become a false god. It is false because first it is not infinite. Oh, how they wished it were so, but it is temporary, as all of life on earth is temporary. It died. Or it left. Or they grew away from it. No matter. The important thing is that it is gone. Yet it is not gone, because it stills controls their lives. It still consumes their energies. It promises them a type of salvation that reads, "If only I could recapture what I lost, then I would be happy." Unfortunately, in the process of idolizing, the persons stuck in grief have "deadened" something else—themselves. They too have stopped living. Not everyone gets this obsessed by grief or has an abnormal mourning experience. Yet to some extent the choice between idolatry and faith is there for all of us each time we face a new loss. To some extent each of us, in every major loss, experiences elements of abnormal grieving. Each loss calls us to give up something that we valued, loved, and needed so dearly. Each loss forces us to emotionally let go of that which we loved. Each loss forces us to let go of the temporary past and move into the future. We may not do so willingly or joyfully, but move into the future we must. For healing and spiritual wholeness lies only in the ever-present future that unfolds before us.

SPIRITUAL HEALTH IN LATER LIFE

As I indicated earlier it is very hard to formulate a definition of spiritual health that will transcend the various stages of the life cycle.

Obviously, what may be spiritually appropriate for an individual at age twenty may be different from what may be spiritually appropriate at age sixty-five. Nevertheless, idolatry offers us a definition of spiritual health that is relevant to every stage of life. At every age people have to choose between faith in the living God and faith in false gods. In bereavement the temptation "to idolize" is acute. To a greater or lesser extent all of us are lured by this natural temptation, augmented by the equally natural defense mechanisms of bereavement.

The spiritually mature person has faith.[8] This faith allows one to grieve, to let go, to release what is lost. Being able to grieve easily and relatively quickly is a very important quality in later life. If we wish to remain psychologically healthy through this difficult period of life, we must be able to grieve well. Faith is an essential ingredient in our ability to grieve. We cannot grieve well without it.

Each time we experience a new loss, we are faced with a choice between faith in a living God that pulls us into the future and faith in false gods that keep us enslaved to the past. In every loss we are tempted "to make idols" out of what was lost. We are tempted in one form or another not to grieve. But by grieving we let go of that past and free ourselves to move into the future. There in the future, God waits for us, longing to make life good again.

Chapter 3

The Loss of Youth

So teach us to number our days that we may get a heart of wisdom.

Ps 90:12

As do all of the losses described in this book, the loss of youth begins gradually, then escalates with each passing year. It is hard to know exactly when certain individuals no longer feel young, when they begin to think of themselves as middle-aged or old or elderly. It is mostly a subjective change, one that can occur at almost any age, but does occur regularly in later life. Usually the first awareness of this loss occurs during the midlife years, between forty and fifty-five, as the individual passes from the first half of life to the second. From then on the loss of youth is a perpetual theme of life.

THE CHANGES OF THE BODY

Usually the first awareness of the loss of youth comes with subtle changes in one's body. At first they are ignored and passed off as momentary limitations. All I need to do is "get back in shape" or "get over this bug that's going around" or "go on a strict diet." But the changes become persistent and in time the signs become clearer, more unmistakable. Their message becomes more and more difficult to avoid.

Can you remember when and where you first realized that you were no longer young? When did you first realize that you were getting older? Perhaps you used to be able to eat pizza and drink beer late at night and sleep like a baby. Then pizza at night started keeping you awake. The digestive tract changed. Did you have a similar experience with coffee? No longer can you have that late night cup of coffee unless you want to be up half the night.

Where else did you first notice it? Perhaps one day you didn't bound up the stairs as you used to. You were winded. Either those stairs got longer or you got older. Probably the latter. Your body has changed. Remember when your muscles first got sore after a little game of softball in the neighborhood? Or how your legs ached when you tried a pirouette? Your body has changed again. Remember when it became harder to study large quantities of material? You just couldn't memorize the way you used to. Your mind had changed—that was the scary one.

I remember the day that my twelve-year-old daughter challenged me to a race back to the beach blanket. That used to be an easy race. I usually had to slow down a bit to make it more exciting. After all, the fun was in the thrill of beating Dad. I remember the day that I stopped pacing myself. She kept getting faster and faster. I kept speeding up, faster and faster, or at least so I thought. I couldn't keep up. I was trying as hard as I could, but the old legs were not moving as fast as they used to. When we both flopped down on the beach blanket, me slightly after her, my diplomatic wife casually remarked, "Well, I guess you are not as young as you used to be." It was a casual remark, a nothing remark, but for me it was one of those moments of sudden clarity. "One day will make you old."[1]

Not only do the inner workings of the body change, but the outward appearance of the body changes as well. Hair begins to show signs of graying or balding or both. Waistlines begin to thicken. Hips widen. Smile lines become permanent. Cheeks droop. Curves aren't where they used to be. Firmness gives way to softness. Of course, we can do more to remake the outward appearance of the body. Trendy clothes, a nice hairstyle, even a face-lift—all do wonders to make one feel youthful and "in step" with the times. It is easy to pretend the body isn't changing.

The decline or change in our appearance is an insidious thing. It strikes so keenly at our vanity. We do need to feel sexually attractive and socially appealing, and to be less so is a change that is difficult to take. When did you notice that people started treating you differently? You flirt with the young girl in the supermarket, and she not only doesn't flirt back, but she has that "I guess I should humor him" look on her face. Oh, how painful! It's walking down the street, thinking you look like a million bucks and secretly wanting to be noticed—and nobody does! How the arrows of fading beauty sting!

All this occurs gradually at first. Then during the later years, bodily changes become a regular occurance. Every year some new change emerges. Every year or so our body tells us again that it has changed and we had better change too. With each passing year the physical alterations become more pronounced and more negative. When we do have an illness or surgery, it now takes longer and longer for our bodies to recover. We used to bounce back within a few days. Now it's a few weeks. The bottom line is that we must make adjustments— adjustments in our lifestyle, in our diet, in our expectations of our- selves physically. To make these adjustments, we must first face the reality of our loss of youth and grieve its passing. Only then, after we have worked through the cognitive and emotional elements, are we motivated to make the necessary behavioral adjustments.

MARKER EVENTS

The loss of youth sneaks up on us emotionally. At a certain level, we know changes are occurring, but we block their full conscious impact. We make minor adjustments and go on pretending. The full awareness of the loss comes to us in what are called "marker events."[2] A marker event is a social occurrence that symbolically marks the passing of time, the transition from one life stage to another. There are many marker events. Almost any occasion can be an eye-opening experience, if the timing is right. One's fortieth birthday is usually such an event. Our child's graduation, first date, or a new driver's license also can be marker events. Perhaps a divorce or a career shift crystal- lizes these changes and makes us fully aware of our loss of youth.

High school class reunions can be weird events. Usually they are dinner dances. A photographer takes an updated picture of the Class of 1963 or whatever. There are lots of decorations and tales from the "good old days" which have gotten better with each telling of the story. Nostalgia drips from the walls. But what is most important are the people—the faces and the names. Most of us are frightened or fascinated to see just how our classmates have changed. Some people look the same—just the same. It is amazing. Others are better. That timid girl with the horn-rimmed glasses—wow! She's now stunningly attractive and socially poised. She's holding court over by the bandstand. Nobody can believe it. And some are worse. Remember the boy who was such a "fox" in high school? Now he's just another middle-aged man with a beer gut, a balding head, and a foul mouth. In some ways he hasn't grown up at all. And with sighs of relief you can hear his former admirers saying, "I'm glad I didn't marry him." Yes, class reunions can be weird events, or better said, events that evoke weird feelings.

I can appreciate why people tend to avoid class reunions. The reunion planners say that it's a stroke of luck if half of the former class members attend. Many people are just too busy. Many have gone on to other relationships and other places. Most just want to avoid the whole thing. Reunions force us to deal with our past, who we were and by implication who we are now. Reunions can be one of those marker events that help us crystallize how far we have—or haven't come. They make us look at ourselves and face the reality that we are no longer young. Most of us come away from class reunions with feelings—relief, fear, fascination, and of course, grief. Reunions can remind us of our lost youth.

We have relatively few socially prescribed marker events in modern urban life.[3] The rituals of former days have faded in the face of the rising tide of secularism and pluralism. The absence of marker events makes it all the easier to avoid dealing with our loss and sorrow. Yet the feelings do sneak up on us. Grief has a way of looking for places to surface. Sometimes when we least expect it or in the seemingly happy events, we are overcome by a sense of sorrow. Then for a moment—perhaps just a moment—we are fully aware of what we have lost.

THE CHANGING CAREER

Individuals who have pursued a lifelong career tend to measure the passing of their lives in terms of work.[4] "Young" and "old" get defined by the career, not by the person. When did you cease to be "a rising star" in your chosen career and start being treated like "a seasoned veteran?" When did they begin to value you for your stability rather than for your vigor, for your loyalty to the company instead of for your creativity, for your stature instead of for your "fresh ideas?" The clues are subtle and differ in each professional group. Professional athletes are old at age thirty. Some people, such as police officers or career military people, can retire after a brief twenty years of service. Executives with aerospace firms are "old" by fifty, because that is the age whereby it is cheaper for the company to hire a younger person just out of college rather than continuing to pay an executive-level salary. Individuals in a trade or skilled labor notice their transition when they can't keep up with the physical demands of their job, when they start to instruct younger people instead of doing it themselves. Doctors, airline pilots, judges, and diplomats seem to reach their peak only after age fifty. These are careers that value wisdom and maturity.

Peter was one of those brilliant young engineers fresh out of MIT when he was sought after by several major construction firms. His doctoral work was in new structural designs for nuclear power plants, a timely and needed subject at the time. His early years with Nash International Construction Company included lots of travel and periods of international residency, supervising the construction of overseas projects. His work was appreciated by the company executives. He even wrote a modest article for a trade journal on his theories of design. As a result, Peter rose rapidly within the ranks of the company and his salary rose correspondingly.

After eighteen years of work, and at the ripe age of forty-eight, Peter was transferred back to the home office, where his work focused more on supervision rather than on implementation. The company had grown some since those early days, and now it needed him back at home supervising the growing number of younger engineers and drafters. At first this was nice, being settled with his family, but after a while, he grew bored and restless.

The awareness began slowly for Peter. There were little signs, such as the younger men referring to him as the "old man" or the way they referred to his once pioneering design theory, as "dated" or the way the CEO fussed over Dave, the newest man in structural work. Peter just felt useless, as though he was a "has-been," as though he had been "put out to pasture." His career was plateauing. There hadn't been a merit increase in years and certainly not an advancement since—well, since he was placed in the home office. Yet, he had to admit to himself that part of him liked this more settled routine. It was easier on his family and on his nerves and part of him liked "fathering" the younger engineers. Yet, part of him also longed for the excitement, the challenge of being on site, seeing the project completed. In his more depressed days he felt as though he was just waiting until retirement. He longed to do something new, something on the cutting edge. That's what led him to make inquiries.

He had to do something. He thought that a new job, perhaps with a new firm, would bring him more satisfaction, more of a challenge. Perhaps a new firm would appreciate him more. That's what he wanted, "to be appreciated." So he put out a few feelers. He was hopeful, upbeat. How could any company not be thrilled to get someone with his experience? He'd have no trouble getting a job, he fantasized, probably a better one than he currently had, and yes, probably one with more opportunity for advancement. Perhaps he could still become a vice president someday.

That was when he heard the word, really *heard* the word—the word "old." It was in the interview with the other firm's officers. Peter was confident, poised, but they were lukewarm, uninterested. He couldn't believe it. A man with his credentials. Then they said it: "Pete, you're a great guy. You've done some great things for this industry—but you're not on the cutting edge right now. We need younger fellows with newer ideas. The business has really become competitive, you know—extremely competitive. It's really not worth it for us to meet your asking salary for someone as old as you are."

Strange, but it helped to hear the word. It hurt, but he felt better in a strange way. In a sense, now he knew. There was no more pretending. Now he felt freer too, freer to go back to Nash and do what he was good at. It was as though he had "let go" of something, and in letting go he was free to be who he really was at this stage of his career.[5]

LOSS OF DREAMS

When we are young we have plenty of dreams. We dream of being rich. We dream of being president of the company, bishop of the diocese, professor at the university, senator in the Congress, or owner and proprietor of The Village Hardware. We dream of having a white house in the suburbs, with a picket fence, three children, and a vacation home in the mountains. We dream of publishing that novel, making that discovery, or patenting that invention. We dream of that special someone who would make us happy. We dream of happiness, achievement and long years ahead. Some of our dreams were pretty unrealistic. Some of them were even illusions. In any case our youth is filled with dreams.

The loss of youth is associated with the loss of dreams and vice versa. One of the signs of getting older, of passing beyond youth, is a painful realization that some of our dreams won't come true. Perhaps we have dreamed too much, fantasized beyond the point of realism. Maybe we have fulfilled some of our dreams—and perhaps the fulfilled dreams did not live up to our expectations. We spent years making a dream come true, only to be disappointed. Or perhaps we are still working for the fulfillment of some dreams. In any event it is becoming increasingly clear, as we get older, that some of our dreams may not be realized. Time is short now. We must let go of the dreams of youth. We must revise our "battle plan."

Judith Viorst, in her book, *Necessary Losses*, describes the many losses of the life cycle that are "necessary," losses that we must experience to grow into the next phase of life. Among these, she describes the loss of dreams and illusions during late middle age this way:

> And we may start to feel that this is a time of always letting go, of one thing after another after another: our waistlines. Our vigor. Our sense of adventure. Our 20/20 vision. Our trust in justice. Our earnestness. Our playfulness. Our dream of being a tennis star, or a TV star, or a senator, or the woman for whom Paul Newman finally leaves Joanne. We give up hoping to read all the books we once had vowed to read, and to go to all the places we'd once vowed to visit. We give up hoping we'll save the world from cancer or from war. We even give up hoping that we will succeed in becoming underweight—or immortal.[6]

Fantasies, dreams, and illusions are subtle things to lose. It is not like losing a home or a spouse or a damaged leg. These are not concrete entities. Nevertheless, they are very real, very powerful, and very determinative to our well-being. Most of us fashion our identities around our dreams. We build a sense of who we are based on our dreams. We plan our life's script around the dreams that we feel we are supposed to fulfill. And our self-esteem rises or falls with the achievement of these dreams. We cannot "live" without dreams. Humans are dreamers. This is why the loss of dreams that comes with later life can invoke such subtle but powerful feelings.

ESCHATOLOGY AND LOSS

As people pass over the midlife point and enter the later years, they report that they have an emerging sense of the limited nature of time. They begin to measure life not by how far they have come, but by how much time they have left.[7] They come to experience life as increasingly limited. In the second half of life the future feels as though it is narrowing; it seems that there are fewer possibilities, fewer options. It is no longer possible to do as much as we wanted to do in our youth. Now we must begin to choose. We must prioritize our goals. "I can't do it all. So what can I do?" asks the person in later years. "How best can I spend these years ahead of me?"

In theological terms this is the clinical experience of eschatology—the awareness of the shortness of the present time.[8] Eschatology is built into the nature of life itself. Life will come to an end. Life is time-limited. In fact, each and every stage of life is time-limited. We often did not feel this sense of time-limitedness when we were youths or young adults. Life seemed more open then, more endless, more filled with possibilities. The problem then was selecting which possibility to achieve first. But in later life, we have a keener sense of the shortness of life in general and in particular of the shortness of our current life stage.

This awareness first emerges into our consciousness during the middle age years and then continues as a regular theme of the later years. Several researchers have noted that the themes of death, dying, and destruction are present in the psyche of the middle-aged person. Daniel J. Levinson, for example, who studied the stages of a man's life writes:

A man in the Mid-Life Transition is troubled by his seemingly imminent death. He is beset even more by the anxiety that he will not be able to make his future better than his past. As he seeks to modify and enrich his life, he has self-doubts ranging in intensity from mild pessimism to utter panic: "Can I make my life more worthwhile in the remaining years? Am I now too old to make a fresh start? Have I become obsolete? What shall I try to do and be for myself, for my loved ones, for my tribe, for humanity?" The worst feeling of all is to contemplate long years of meaningless existence without youthful passions, creative effort or social contribution.[9]

Levinson has described so well the eschatological crisis. The awareness of death and the shortness of life raises questions of meaningfulness and worthwhileness. These questions lead people to reflect on and re-examine their lives and their goals. The dreams, illusions, and plans of youth must be revised. In later life the individual may have to "let go" of some of the dreams of his or her youth. The youthful dreams must now be tempered with the realisms of the later years.

April always wanted to be a ballet dancer, but an early marriage, several children and odd working hours prevented all of that. When her daughters were old enough for lessons, however, she encouraged them to take ballet. The youngest seemed especially motivated. For many years, April shared in and through her child's accomplishments. As she approached forty she began to be restless about her unfulfilled dream. "It's now or never," she thought. "I'll never be a ballerina at this point in my life, but I still want to learn; I still want to dance. What have I got to lose? I'm not getting any younger." So she enrolled in classes alongside her teenage daughter. In recent years the two of them have danced in several community productions separately and together. According to April, she has never been happier.

Life in the later years has this sense of eschatology about it, a keener awareness of the shortness of the present age. While this awareness first comes to us during the midlife years, it is not limited to those years. It is a theme that permeates the whole second half of life. In the early 1990s, Phillip Berman and Connie Goldman interviewed famous people, all over sixty years old, people mostly from the field of entertainment and the arts, on the subject of aging, more specifically, their aging. The resulting book, *The Ageless Spirit*, is a collection of reflections and observations on aging from these well-known people. What interested me most, however, were not the individual reflections, as inspiring as they were, but the overall conclusions compiled by the editors after completing and reflecting upon these lengthy, and, at times, intense interviews. Chief among their observations was this: "As Time diminishes, its preciousness increases."[10] The editors, reflecting on the common themes, continue, "Time, which represents the gift of life, is no longer a commodity to be squandered thoughtlessly on vain and empty pursuits." Seniors or people at any stage in the second half of life, have this sense that time is short, and in growing short, it becomes so precious.

When people become fully aware of this new reality, this shortness of time, they respond in a variety of ways. Some people respond to this awareness with despair. Some respond with panic, others, with denial. Still others are motivated to redeem the time they have left and to make the most of it. The latter approach, which is more healthy psychologically and spiritually, is possible only if a person has grieved the loss of his or her youth.

SOCIETY'S PERVASIVE INFLUENCE

Our experience of the loss of youth is influenced in large measure by social norms and attitudes. Being old is partially a social phenomenon. You are "old" when others tell you that you are old and you are still "young" if you behave the way others say a young person should behave.[11] Social roles and expectations are subtle pressures. I remember that during my younger years as a family therapist, I took pride in my ability to work effectively with adolescents. It seemed as though I could relate well to them, and many teens confirmed this self-perception during those years. Some ten or so years later, however, I remember being aware how much more often I seemed to side emotionally with the parents. I was sympathizing more with the parents' frustration than with the teen's rebellion. (It was no coincidence that I was a parent myself now.) Then one day it was confirmed. Susie was a sixteen-year-old client who announced after the first session that she didn't like me as a counselor. She wanted someone her own age, someone who could understand her. I was put in my place—in more ways than one.

Each society defines "young" and "old" in its own terms and gives to these terms its own connotations. In American society, "old" carries a negative connotation and "young" has a positive flavor. Old is considered obsolete, useless, out of date. Old appliances are thrown out. Old clothes are discarded. Old technology is not cost efficient and so it is replaced. This is a disposal society. When it gets old, throw it away. Little wonder then that older people feel as though they are being thrown away too. Their advice is not sought after. They are isolated from the mainstream of society. They are now useless, the "discards" of society.

America is a youth-worshiping culture. The mass media reflects that. We love our young ideas, our fresh faces, our beautiful bodies. Progress has also been our collective idol. If it's new, it must be better. Yes, we worship progress. What we have not valued by comparison is maturity, tradition, roots, aged wisdom. Perhaps as the percentage of older people in the population increases, as it is expected to over the next fifty years, we will see a greater shift toward a more balanced picture of young and old. But for the moment, the connotations of the word "old" are still largely negative.

It also seems to be a well-established fact that there is in this society a kind of ageism, which Alex Comfort defines as "the notion that people cease to be people, cease to be the same people or become people of a distinct and inferior kind, by virtue of having lived a specific number of years. . . ."[12] This ageism, like its cousins racism and sexism, results in overt and covert acts of discrimination, bias and stereotyping. I suspect that ageism is the flip side of our society's obsession with youth. Both features, the ageism and the idolatry of youth, are products of our collective denial.[13] We deny that we are aging. We deny that we are no longer young. In countless ways this society encourages that denial and we are all willing players in one form or another. How then is it possible for reasonable people to recognize, much less grieve, their loss of youth? At best it is difficult. At worst it never happens, and most people, when they finally realize that they are old, slip into a chronic state of despair and therein live out the remainder of their lives.

FINDING POSITIVE MEANINGS FOR "OLD"

Ultimately, of course, "old" and "young" are not fixed commodities. There is no prescribed age that dictates when one is old.[14] Indeed, there are social pressures, but ultimately "old" and "young" are subjective experiences. We can be old way before our years and we can be "young at heart" way beyond our years. We have all known people in both camps. If we are to experience healthy later years, we must transform the connotations attached to the words "old" and "young." We must, as Levinson says, "find positive meanings to being 'older'" and integrate the young and old within us.[15] Part of the grieving we do for our lost youth is a coming to terms with the word "old". . . . and with all the labels that attempt to limit us. Successful grieving will include an embracing and accepting of these words and a transforming of them into positive images for us.

One of the barriers to this kind of transformation of the word "old" resides in the model of aging that most of us have in our minds. The prevailing model of aging is what is called the "Rise-Peak-Decline" model. This model, sometimes called the "low-high-low model," sees people growing throughout the first half of life and reaching a peak of development around midlife and then spending the remainder of their lives in a long slow decline toward death. That's a pretty depressing view of the human journey! No wonder no one wants to enter the second half of life. Some evidence supports this view, of course. Certainly in physical terms, we do grow, reach a peak, and then slowly decline. Yet, when we view humans from a holistic perspective, we must agree with pastoral counselor William M. Clements that "The low-high-low scheme of viewing developmental reality is an illusion."[16] How do we account for such people as Winston Churchill, Albert Schweitzer, and Immanuel Kant, all of whom had their most productive and creative years late in life? Such people as these do not decline in later years. On the contrary, they continue to grow well into "old age" and probably right up to death's door. We might say that they end their lives at the peak of their spiritual development.

If we are to live the later years of our lives in psychological and spiritual health, we must revise our thinking about aging itself. We must realize that "the upward curve," as ethicist Charles E. Curran calls it, can and should continue throughout our entire life span.[17] We do not have to decline mentally or spiritually. On the contrary, we should look forward to old age the way we looked forward to our senior year of college, with anticipation and excitement for a time that will be the climax of our journey.[18] After many years of preparation, we are finally "going to put it all together." The later years can be a time of rich experience, deep relationships, and spiritual maturity. If these years are to be such, however, we must transform the word "old" from a negative image into a positive one. Grieving our lost youth inevitably includes this kind of transforming.

EMBRACING THE PRESENT

The loss of youth is one of those necessary losses. We must deal with it and grieve it, if we are to go on with our lives, if we are to accept and even embrace who we are now. People have varieties of ways of coping or failing to cope with their loss of youth.

At age forty-three, James was hardly an old man, but he felt like it. He was keenly aware of all of the little signs of aging. Each tiny change in his appearance panicked him. He didn't want to be old and didn't think that he had to be. So he worked out with weights, wore designer clothes, put a rinse on his hair, drove a sports car, and delighted in the looks of the younger women at his office. His rationalization was, "Salesmen have to maintain a young image. People don't want to deal with an old man." Maintaining his youth was linked with maintaining his job, thus giving even greater importance to the obsession to stay young.

From the vantage point of grief dynamics, James was denying the emerging loss of his youth. His feelings of sorrow frightened him. Too much of his worth and identity was tied up in being youthful. So he fled from his feelings, in the opposite direction, idolizing his lost youth. That worked well enough for a while, but with each passing year, James' defense mechanisms became all the more silly. By the time he was fifty-three years old, the tight pants and hip style weren't cute. Instead of flirting with him, the younger women were now feeling sorry for him. Sex appeal turned to pity.

Let me suggest another version of a person denying the loss of youth. Patty first came to me for marriage counseling. She had been married for almost seventeen years, but increasingly she felt bored with the relationship. She complained that there was no excitement, no passion, no romance in her life.

"Oh, he's a great guy," she would say, "and a great father, but I don't know if I really love him anymore. I love him, but I'm not in love with him. Do you know what I mean?"

"Not really," I responded. "Explain it to me."

"When we were younger and first in love, everything was exciting. He was so handsome, so sexy. We just couldn't stay away from each other. And we'd talk hours on end, sometimes until three in the morning. We just wanted to be together always."

"It sounds as though you are grieving for your lost romance."

"Sometimes I just want to run away," she continued. "I want to start over, maybe move up north. Make a new start. The kids can make it on their own. And Jack can easily find someone else. He's a good man. I have this deep urge to start over, before . . . ."

"Before what?"

". . . . before it's too late."

The situations and feelings of Patty and James are so common that they are almost caricatures. Most counselors and clergypersons have talked with many people caught in these same dynamics. Both of these cases are, in my view, examples of individuals seeking to avoid facing their loss of youth. James felt it most sharply in terms of his appearance and physique. Patty felt it more in the relationship area where she longed for the lost romance of younger days. They both attempted to deny their loss in one form or another, to avoid their feelings, and even to flee from their own inner pain. James never seemed to deal openly with his feelings and eventually became an object of pity, not envy. Patty dealt more openly with her feelings and eventually worked out her grief. Coupled with marital counseling, she was able to revitalize her marriage.

Theologically, I suggest that both James and Patty have made youth into a false god. The god of youth is a very popular idol in America. There is plenty of encouragement for and money in the idolization of youth. James has many people who want to sell him a product or a service that will help him deny his aging. Patty can wallow in soap operas and romance novels if she wants to worship at the altar of young love all day. Neither of them will grow psychologically or spiritually because of their allegiance to the god of youth. They will continue to believe that true happiness, i.e., salvation, lies in returning to the past, to something that is essentially lost.

Persons caught in this kind of idolatry refuse psychologically to be their age. In a sense they are defying God's rule. God has intended everything that is alive to age. By refusing to mourn their youth, by refusing to even acknowledge the reality of loss, they are also refusing to accept God's reign. It is as if they are saying psychologically that "I am the creator, not God. I reject God's creation." They cannot imagine that life can be good in the future or even in the present. For them, salvation seems to be found in going backward, not forward.

At age seventy-three Paul Tournier, the Swiss physician and popular Christian writer of the last generation, was asked to reflect on aging and old age.[19] In reflecting on what constitutes successful aging, he focused in on the theme of acceptance. If we are able to age well, he suggested, we must be able "to accept life in its entirety." Part of this acceptance, for Tournier, is accepting who and what we are at every stage of our life. He writes:

> To play the old man when one is young or the young man when one is old; to behave like a single person when one is married; to put on masculine manners when one is a woman; to affect love for a father whom one hates or to pretend to embrace when one is not—all this leaves behind it an ineradicable malaise, the feeling that one is in disharmony with oneself, with the truth about oneself. There is in the human heart a need for truth which one can indeed betray, but cannot get rid of.[20]

From Tournier's words, I want to emphasize the word "acceptance," as a powerful theme of what it means to be psychologically healthy in the context of aging. Acceptance means accepting the age or stage of life we are currently in. It means being what we are. Acceptance is the opposite of denial. Denial rejects the present and wants the past. Acceptance embraces the present and looks forward to the future. This is another good definition of spiritual health that would be applicable to any age. It is also, interestingly enough, the fifth and final stage of Kübler-Ross' stages of anticipatory grief.[21] Her stages begin with denial and end, if possible, with acceptance. The person of faith or maturity accepts life and his or her current life stage, even if that life stage is the last. Acceptance is a good word for the ultimate goal of all grief work. If we do our grief work well, we come to accept reality.

The loss of youth does not happen all at once. We tend to notice it first at midlife, but the issue stays with us throughout the later years.

The loss of youth is a gradual and persistent experience, and periodically over the years we will probably need to pause and identify this loss again and again. We will feel its pain most as marker events. At those times, we must, as Eugene C. Bianchi suggests:

> Seriously enter into the experience of the sands slipping away in the hourglass of our lives. This discomforting feeling of the unstoppable dimming of the light, the numbering of our breaths, must be embraced until it hurts.[22]

Grieving is indeed painful, but it is the only way to health or "acceptance." So when those moments come, take time to grieve. Allow yourself some time and space to cry a little. For only in doing so can we again embrace the present.

As we discuss the other losses of the later years in later chapters, we would do well to remember this definition of mental and spiritual health as acceptance. We should not "borrow from the future" by living in fear of the next life stage. Neither should we live in the past by "idolizing" the life stage just completed. Live fully in the present. Enjoy it. Embrace it. Look for God there. However, to fully embrace the present, we must regularly let go of the past, and one of the most significant losses that we must periodically let go of is the loss of our youth.

Chapter 4

The Loss of Family

And his mother said to him, "Son, why have you treated us
so?". . . . And he said to them, "How is it that you sought me?
Did you not know that I must be in my Father's house?"

Lk 2:48-49

We spend the middle years of adult life in building. We build a
family, a career, a home, and place in the community. It is a time for
planting roots deep into the soil of our psyches. We build memories
that last a lifetime. We form deep emotional attachments to one
another. The later half of life, however, is a time when what has been
built up gradually begins to dissolve. One by one (or, sometimes, all at
once) we will let go of family, career, and home. This chapter will
focus on the loss of family, which begins as the children progressively
become more autonomous, then independent, and finally leave the
family nest to lead their own lives and start their own families. Eventually, there are just the two of you again . . . or sometimes just one of
you. The empty nest.

A COMPLEXITY OF EMOTIONS

I do not know too many parents who do not cognitively acknowledge that they want their children to be independent, autonomous
adults. That is the ultimate goal of all parenting. Emotionally, however,
parents may have other feelings, some conscious, some unconscious,
that influence how they handle their personal loss of family. Emotionally, it may be difficult to let go of children, because this loss involves
so many other issues. Letting go of children may mean:

- The end of my primary identity as parent.
- That I cannot control my children anymore, which in turn may mean that I am a failure.
- My spouse and I no longer have any glue to hold us together.
- A deep sense of disappointment over how the children have turned out.
- That I cannot protect them from harm any longer and must risk their ultimate loss.
- I am getting older and all of the implications therein.
- I am no longer needed, or important.

Thus, the process of letting go of our children gets complicated. It may get contaminated with other issues and feelings. The grief is not pure.

Irene was a mother of three children. The first two seemed to grow up reasonably well in spite of the divorce that split up the family. It helped that they were into their preteens by the time the family separated. But Jimmy was younger than the rest by six years. He was Irene's baby, her desperate attempt to save the marriage by having a third child. Having Jimmy did not save the marriage, but it did create a strong and enmeshed bond between Irene and this child. Jimmy was six when his father left. From that point on, Irene raised him alone as best she could. Jimmy was a handful to raise—a very bright child, a bit precocious, and he had a quick temper even from an early age. In addition, he got used to being on his own, since his mother was gone a lot at work and on dates. She was always hoping to find Jimmy a father to replace the one that she blamed herself for taking away. Jimmy, of course, never liked any of the men his mother brought home, and made his views plain enough by his behavior.

As Jimmy grew older, the conflicts with his mother intensified. Irene didn't like his smart mouth, his defiant attitude, and his growing independence. She felt rejected by this child, "her baby" to whom she had given so much. He more or less ran wild in his early teens, and any attempt by Irene to put restrictions on him was met with outrage, defiance, and running-away behaviors. Jimmy was becoming a master at manipulating his mother, a situation that she allowed because she couldn't say no.

Eventually Irene fell in love with another man and remarried, all of which necessitated that she move to another community to join her new mate. It seemed most appropriate at this time, given Jimmy's incorrigible behavior, to have him live with his natural father, who had by now also remarried. This would give Jimmy and his father time to get to know each other again. This arrangement worked for a while. Then Jimmy began to misbehave at his dad's house too. When his father attempted to place restrictions on Jimmy, he would call his mother and "run away" to her house. She, of course, couldn't say no and would take him in. "Jimmy and I are so close. . . . and he has had such a hard time of it," she would rationalize to herself. Sometime later Jimmy would miss his friends and go back to Dad's. Jimmy went back and forth like this several times, playing one household against the other.

The issue reached crisis proportions when the local sheriff arrested Jimmy for selling drugs, and the juvenile division officer recommended hospitalization for Jimmy for a brief period to get control of his behavior and his drug problem. Irene refused. "That's too drastic," she replied. "Jimmy is not that kind of kid. All he needs is love and attention." Irene couldn't or wouldn't face the reality that Jimmy had become a criminal, that he was out of control and that he had a drug problem. At a deeper level Irene was denying that Jimmy was grown up, that she couldn't protect him any longer and that her "little boy" was gone. Irene's inability to let go actually prevented Jimmy from getting the help he needed. Eventually, he ran afoul of the law again, and this time he was forced to get help through a period of confinement in a state youth camp.

My point in telling this story is to illustrate how complicated the process of letting go of one's children can be. Besides the obvious feelings of sorrow, many other issues can get tangled up in the process, issues that usually have to do with the parent's needs and pathologies. Irene's difficulty in letting go of Jimmy expressed itself early in the way she failed to discipline the boy. She couldn't deal with the pain of loss, of letting go of that last child, the last vestige of her motherhood and family. When Irene attempted to say no, Jimmy's defiance hooked her fear of losing him. Her difficulty was compounded by the false meanings she attached to this situation. It meant failure as a parent. Coupled with her perceived failure as a marriage partner, her self-worth couldn't risk another failure.[1] Because she could not deal with all this, she distorted the parent-child relationship, and her effectiveness as a parent was greatly diminished.

THE PROCESS CHARACTER OF THIS LOSS

The loss of family, like most losses in later life, is experienced as a gradual process. Actually parents can start losing their children, emotionally and socially, fairly early in life. In a sense, parenthood is or should be a lifelong process of "letting go." The process accelerates when the children move into the early adolescent period with its natural surge toward autonomy. Increasingly children in this period move away from dependency. They start making some of their own decisions without relying on or consulting with their parents. They start valuing the opinions of peers more than those of their parents. All the signs are there, if we notice them.

Do you remember how you felt when your young teenage daughter first kept a secret from you? The locked diary? The secret letter to a friend at camp? Now there is a part of her life that you do not share. Some parents find this secrecy threatening. Others ride with it as natural development. Remember too, the time perhaps a little later, when your son first decided that attending a family event wasn't as important to him as attending an event with his friends? He chose peers over family. How did you feel? Did you allow his decision or enforce your will that he go with the family? It is hard to know how much freedom to allow a young adult without losing family unity. Embedded in this issue is how you, as a parent, feel about the growing distance between you and your child.

As teenagers grow older into late adolescence, their independence grows as well. Now they are literally gone more. Perhaps they drive now and so they spend more time away from home. More and more they manage their own money, choose their own clothes, select their own friends, form their own priorities. In addition, the culture fosters the growing distance between teenager and parents by creating a teen subculture. The youth culture has its own fashions, its own language and its own music, all of which reinforces the adolescent's natural urge to be different, to be autonomous. At times it seems as though our children are becoming a different species. We don't recognize them, much less communicate with them. That's frustrating and frightening. We want them to be "like us," but we also want them to be their own person. Which side of this dilemma do we push?

Some parents do not encourage autonomy in their children. They perceive their adolescent's emerging autonomy as an approaching loss. They are frightened by their feelings of loss, so they resist the change in subtle and not so subtle ways. All of this makes "leaving home" a much more difficult and even traumatic experience for the family than it might otherwise have been, and in some tragic cases causes a bitterness between parent and child that is never repaired. Psychiatrist Roger L. Gould reminds us of the inevitability of growth when he writes:

> If we "stonewall" against changing and insist that our main role is to be their parents, we can force their changes into less healthy but nevertheless necessary expression. Like the flow of a powerful river, the need to grow can only be diverted, never totally dammed.[2]

Other parents, of course, do encourage autonomy in their teenage children. Such parents have prepared themselves well for the eventual loss of family and accept its gradual coming with grace and patience. Such parents, in my view, have done their grief work. They have faced their own feelings, and by so doing they are better able to pass through this transition and better able to facilitate their children's passage. Autonomy comes gradually, and so grieving should come gradually as well. If autonomy and "letting go" both occur in parallel steps, then each step toward autonomy will be one that both parent and child are ready for.[3]

For Christian parents the task can be both more difficult and filled with more resources. Pastoral theologian Herbert Anderson comments on the nature of love and parenthood for Christians when he says:

> The process of leaving home is often as painful as it is necessary . . . . For parents, the fundamental task is to act out the conviction that loving means letting go. The parental love that lets go and sends children forth to serve in the world parallels the love of God in Christ. For Christian parents, baptism has been a sign from the beginning that our children already belong to God.[4]

Remembering that our children belong to God is a helpful barrier against "making idols" out of children or out of the nuclear family. It is also a way of encouraging us to grieve "in advance" the eventual loss of our children as children. We must always remember that our children will not be children forever. Yet, effective parents are not just those who grieve well, but those who know how to balance loving and grieving, holding close and letting loose, restricting and liberating. Both elements are important.

AMBIVALENT FEELINGS

Like few other losses, the loss of family carries a mixture of positive and negative feelings. Talking to parents who are largely through this transition reveals the primary feelings of nostalgia and relief.

I was sitting with Harold and Jane who were sharing with me some of their feelings now that their child-rearing years are largely over. I asked them to show me their family albums in which they have pictures of their children from birth on. Most parents have several of these albums filled with pictures.[5] As we thumbed through the pages, the pictures brought back wonderful memories. Often, a particular picture would trigger a story or two. They would say, "Remember . . ."

> . . . when Susan first learned to ride a bicycle? I can still see you holding on to the rear seat, running along beside her, as she wobbled down the sidewalk.
> . . . the time we bought a puppy for Daniel's fourth birthday? We hid it in the laundry room overnight and it cried like a baby. You ended up sleeping with it.
> . . . how scared I was when Susy first started driving on her own? Gosh, we thought for sure we would hear from the police or the hospital within the hour.
> . . . when Danny was in that hiking accident and we spent all night at the hospital, waiting to see if he was going to pull through? And what did he say when he woke up, "Where's the ice cream?"
> . . . the year you coached Brandon's Little League team? Now that was an experience! The screaming parents. The innocent kids. And the day that Brandon hit the home run that won the game. Those were great times.
> . . . how Susan looked on her wedding day? How beautiful. How grown up. I will never forget that day as long as I live. Let me show you Susy's wedding pictures.[6]

Almost every parent has memories like these. It is not too hard to get most post-parenting couples to talk about their memories of their family years. Even the trying times and the scary times don't seem so bad from the perspective of the later years. Even the rough years seem wonderful. Most people can easily identify their feelings of nostalgia for the family years.

Yet, within the same breath and certainly within the same conversation, the couple also talked about their feelings of freedom. I asked them, "Would you do it again? Would you like to have a family back—perhaps another child?"

"Nope, not on your life!" they announced. "Too much responsibility. Too much worry. We are too old for that now. God was wise to give children to younger parents. You have the energy for them then, and the time and the patience. Now it's a relief just to have them grown up."

Jane was especially thankful not to have children around. "Those were great years," she said, "but since then I have developed my own flower shop. The shop has been something that I always wanted to do. I began it when Brandon was still in high school, and now it's going great guns. I wouldn't have time for a family now, even if I wanted one—and I don't." Many women can relate to Jane's situation. It's nice having the free time that the empty-nest years allow. Now there is time to develop a career, travel, or enjoy that often neglected hobby.

Most of us can identify with these common emotions: nostalgia and relief or freedom. Other post-parenting adults may have strong, more extreme versions of these emotions. They may long deeply for the lost family and correspondingly don't feel very positive about the empty-nest years. They still live in and through the lives of their children. Perhaps they interfere with the lives of their adult children. Perhaps they are still trying to mother or father—trying to control, trying to be needed. They feel as if they are not needed anymore, and that's painful.

At the other extreme, some parents may have bitter feelings about their children's departure. Perhaps their children did not turn out so well. They are not only relieved that parenting is over, but angry and resentful that it didn't turn out better. They feel that their children owe them more—more respect, more help, more something. "The children just took, took, took," they complain, "and never, not once, said 'thank you.'" Have you met such parents?

The feelings we experience concerning the loss of family can be and usually are very ambivalent. They certainly include nostalgia, relief, freedom, and perhaps anger—a collection of emotions that can best be understood as a grief process.

THE WOUNDED PARENTS

We all have dreams for our children. We want them to be happy, well-adjusted. We dream that they will achieve importance. We dream of their careers, their marriages, their accomplishments. Sometimes we dream dreams for them that are really our own unfulfilled dreams.[7] We live our lives over again in them. That is dangerous. We also have more specific expectations for our children. We expect them to follow our morals, our family standards, our dictates regarding grades, behavior, and the like. What happens when they do not fulfill our dreams or follow our expectations? In fact, they reject our wishes in large part. This can be a powerful and painful loss.

Betty and Bob were very religious people. Bob had been raised in a Christian home with a strict moral code. Betty had been raised in a broken home, but wanted to do better by her children. They thought that they had given their oldest daughter, Mary, everything that a child could want or need. This included not only material things, but also affection, family stability, and proper religious training. It seemed as though Mary flowered in this environment. She was a nice, well-behaved child who never did much without consulting her parents. In her teens, she became more independent than her age merited, but her parents always trusted her. Actually, there were many signs of trouble, but her parents did not see them. So it really came as a shock to them when she ran away from home the summer before her senior year in high school.

The couple found out two days later that Tom, an eighteen-year-old recent high school graduate, also had left home the same day. And they found out from Tom's stepfather that Mary and Tom had been going together for the past six months. That was the real shocker! Why did Mary hide this from them? What else might be going on? Their minds imagined the worst. Bob's shock turned to anger: "How could she do this to us?" He wanted to disown his daughter on the spot. Betty's reaction was more guilt-oriented: "What did I do wrong? Why didn't she come to us? Why won't she contact us now?"

The couple heard from Mary some time later. She was living with Tom on a ranch of sorts in a nearby state. Bob wanted to go there immediately and force her to come home, but Mary threatened to run away farther if he came after her. The parents could do nothing but wait. Conversations by telephone and letters occurred, and piece by piece, more of the story unfolded of how Mary fell in love with Tom but couldn't confide in her parents who she knew would disapprove of him; of how she felt alienated from church and the family's moral code; and of how she just wanted to "have fun" and "be on her own" for a while. The parents felt rejected by their daughter's communications. Their frustration turned to anger and depression. They felt helpless. For the first time in their life Mary was out of their sight, out of their reach—to both control and to aid. They were afraid and angry.

Four months passed. Bob and Betty had their hands full trying to explain this situation to their younger children, to Mary's church friends, and to the extended family. It was a painful time. Through conversations with her daughter (Bob refused to talk to her), Betty felt that part of the story was being concealed. Betty reflected that Mary sounded more unsure of herself in recent weeks. This weighed heavily on Bob and Betty. Then one Saturday, Bob announced that he had had enough of this and decided to take matters into his own hands. He drove all day and night to the place where he suspected that Mary lived. Upon his arrival, he found Mary living in a commune-type arrangement, but there was no Tom to be found. He had recently left, but not without leaving his mark—Mary was eight months pregnant. Bob was able to persuade his daughter to come home with him, at least for the baby's sake.

Mary's attitude toward her parents did not improve much at home. She was hostile toward them and resented their attempts to help her as ploys to make her stay home, "like I was a little kid or something." The couple couldn't understand why Mary resented them so much. They were "only trying to help." Fortunately, they were able to get Mary into some counseling and eventually that personal counseling evolved into family therapy. This process helped all of the family co-exist during the period surrounding the baby's birth.

The relationship between Mary and her parents never really improved until years later. And today, some ten years later, they all agree that they have an excellent relationship. The key factors that facilitated the healing of their relationship were Mary's experience of being a mother herself and her parents coming to terms with their own feelings of loss and resentment toward their daughter. Concerning the second factor, the family continued in counseling long after Mary dropped out. Their primary task during that period of counseling was to work on the terrible sense of loss that they felt about Mary. They believed Mary had "thrown her life away." She was given everything and gave it up for a pigpen. Bob and Betty couldn't understand it or accept it. They had such wonderful dreams for Mary. She could have been anything she wanted—a doctor, a missionary, a teacher. Through counseling they were forced to acknowledge that they were in a prolonged grief process, not for Mary per se, but the idealized Mary of their dreams. Perhaps the idealized Mary had become an idolized Mary, an idol that promised a kind of false salvation for Bob and Betty. Letting go of that idol allowed them to experience grief for that idealized daughter, thus paving the way for a new, healthier relationship with their "real" adult daughter.

VARIATIONS ON THE THEME

These are times in which the normal or typical nuclear family has given way to various other types of family constellations. We now have more single-parent families, more serial marriages, more childless couples, and so on. The theme of family loss has many variations. Let's look at some examples.

Donna is currently a sixty-four-year-old single woman, who has always been timid and dependent. Her husband walked out on her some twenty years earlier, but her four children have continued to be involved in her life. Two of the children continued to live with her in the family home well into their twenties. Then one of the older girls, following her divorce, moved back in with Mom, bringing her two-year-old with her. Donna has not experienced the loss of her family yet. She has always been "Mom" in one form or another. She probably will not really go through this transition until she is almost seventy and then it will probably be a welcome relief.

Melvin was a father of four children, ages eight to sixteen, when he and his wife divorced. It was a very bitter divorce, partly because Linda quickly married the man that she had been having an affair with during her marriage to Melvin. All four children decided to remain living with their mother in the family home with the new stepfather. Melvin tried to keep up with the visitations with his children as regularly as he could, but over the years his visitations grew more infrequent. The older children had busy schedules that left little time for Dad, and Mel's company began to ask him to travel more often (partly because they knew that he was unencumbered with family now). Six years passed. Melvin became more dissatisfied with his life. He was depressed and very lonely in spite of his girlfriend's affection. He could never pinpoint the problem until his oldest daughter got married and he could not attend the wedding because he had to be out of town. Then he began to realize how much he had missed out on during the past few years. He wasn't there to see Paul drive or see Esther's first date or Timmy's soccer games. He missed all that. He had been cheated out of fatherhood. Mel's loss of family was very painful.

Jerry had two families. His first marriage was early in his life and resulted in four children. His first wife died of cancer when the children were approaching young adulthood. He coped as a single parent for five years, seeing the oldest two children through high school. It was hard to get over the death of his wife, and in spite of a modest social life, he never got serious about anyone. His wife was still there in the faces and mannerisms of the two oldest girls. As they finished high school and one went to college and the other got married, it was almost as though he was losing Michelle (his wife) all over again. Yet, he also experienced a sense of freedom. He subsequently entered a relationship with a woman who was twelve years his junior. Elizabeth and he soon married and she brought one child to this new marriage. Jerry and Elizabeth then had a baby of their own within a year. Now the household included "mine, yours, and ours." About the time that Jerry finished with one family, he started another. His experience of the loss of family was prolonged and double barreled.

What becomes clear from these sample vignettes is that "family" means more than the mere presence of children. Family means everything we associate with home and family life. When we lose family, we lose a home, an identity, and, maybe most of all, a way of life.[8]

THE PHYSIOLOGICAL COMPONENT

The loss of family, as described in this book, is primarily a sociopsychological process. However, for women, a clear physical change also is associated, at least symbolically, with the loss of family. That physical change is, of course, menopause. Menopause occurs when the monthly reproductive cycle ceases. In Western societies, it usually occurs between ages forty-eight to fifty-one. For a woman, it is the loss of fertility, the final realization that she can no longer bear a child.

A woman's reaction to this loss can vary from relief to sadness. For some women this change of life is welcome. They are glad to be done with the inconvenience and discomfort of menstrual cycles. For others menopause is experienced as a confirmation and an intensification of what they are already experiencing interpersonally—the loss of children, the advent of the empty nest. When these two processes occur at approximately the same time, they can reinforce and intensify each other. The "drying up" of a woman's monthly flow can symbolize "the dying" of her motherly role, her identity, and the loss of family. For women who have never given birth it can represent an even more powerful loss, the loss of this ability forever.

It is interesting to observe that menopause is often referred to as "the change of life." This popular description of menopause is filled with more truth than we might otherwise admit, particularly when it is associated with the loss of family. For there may be more that is changing here than just a woman's biochemistry. At about the same time, a woman is dealing with the passage of her children from childhood to adulthood and correspondingly the passage of her role from mother to friend. The physiological process and the interpersonal process may mirror each other. With this "change of life," the adult woman enters a new life stage filled with new potential and new possibilities.

The so-called male menopause is usually described as an increased frequency of male sexual impotence and/or a declining or altering of male sexuality. This change, if it really is an identifiable event, is more gradual than the women's change of life. The "male menopause" is also more of a psychological change than a physiological one. Psychologically, it is experienced as a loss of vitality and a loss of youth. The man's experience of increased sexual impotence raises feelings of loss, vulnerability, and inadequacy more often associated with the typical male midlife crisis (see Chapter 3) than with the loss of family passage.

THE PASSAGE TO THE EMPTY NEST

The post–child-rearing stage of life is popularly known as the empty-nest period. In the more formal literature, the empty nest period is defined as the interval in a couple's life between the time that the last child leaves home and a first spouse dies. As we view the human life cycle from a historical perspective, we note that this stage of life has actually lengthened with the advent of better health habits and modern medical procedures. In *The Bonus Years*, Thomas B. Robb notes that the older couple today will spend two-thirds as much time in the empty-nest period as they did in child rearing. In 1890, the death of the first spouse occurred on average two years before the completion of the parental role, whereas in 1950, this event occurred approximately fourteen years after the end of the child-rearing period.[9] What this means is that we have more time than ever before because the home is probably empty of children, at least our immediate children. The heavy responsibilities of parenthood are probably finished. Probably more money is available now than ever before in our lives. Hopefully, no limiting health problems have arisen yet. This stage of life, then, can be one of the most creative, productive, and stable in the lives of individuals or couples if we can adapt well to the loss of family.

Robert C. Peck, who has specialized in the study of the personality of older adults, has attempted to describe the psychological changes that need to occur in an individual if he or she is to pass through the later years of life in good psychological health. In that regard, he introduced the term "cathectic flexibility," which, according to him, is one crucial feature of successful aging. Cathectic flexibility is a type of "emotional flexibility" or "the capacity to shift emotional investments from one person to another, and from one activity to another."[10] Peck argues that if we are to age well, we must develop this ability to let go of past emotional investments and reinvest ourselves in new attachments. Translated: one must learn to grieve well in the sense of letting go of emotional attachments. The opposite of this, "cathectic impoverishment," occurs when a person gradually loses love objects, but does not replace them with new attachments. Gradually the person becomes more and more emotionally impoverished. Erik H. Erikson's term, "stagnate" comes to mind as well. There are fewer and fewer "things" that the person cares about. Without caring the older person stagnates.

This concept can obviously apply to any and all of the losses during the later years of life. However, nowhere is it more applicable than as it pertains to the loss of family and the transition into the "creative years."[11] Robert Peck placed this crisis in the middle years of the adult's life. Persons who can be flexible regarding the loss of their children and their parental roles, are able to form new attachments that will enrich this period of their lives. Others who are emotionally rigid cannot let go and will remain stuck in the past, never to find the full potential of the empty-nest period. How well the loss of family is handled then significantly colors how creative or uncreative the empty-nest period will really be.

Like nothing else, the loss of family signals the loss of a clearly defined and widely accepted social role, i.e., being a mother or father. The loss of this role seems to be especially hard on people who have anchored their self-worth and identity in parenting and the parental role. Such people, as we would expect from the attachment theory of grief, would have a more difficult time transitioning into the empty-nest stage of their life cycle. The more emotional attachment or meaning that a person places on that which is lost, the more difficult it is, generally, for that individual to transition.[12] The loss of family creates a type of mini crisis of meaning or identity crisis for the overly invested parent. Not only are there questions of identity, "Who am I now that I am no longer an active parent?" but also questions of worth and meaning, "What is my worth?" If a woman or a man is to move through this passage well, she or he must wrestle with these questions of meaning and identity, and find in this transition a new, broader, and perhaps a richer definition of self.

FROM CHILDREN TO FRIENDS

Unlike many other losses in later life, the loss of family offers us a wonderful opportunity for a new relationship with our adult children.

In this sense the loss of family is a necessary loss, if one is to find new, improved, and more mature relationships with one's children, spouse, and the world in general. Many post-parental adults speak fondly of the relationship they now have with their adult children, relationships characterized often as friendships. Such relationships are not possible until the loss of family experience is passed through, by both parents and children.

Many parents see their children as extensions of themselves or as their possessions, or as the fulfillment of their unfulfilled lives. These are all potentially destructive attitudes to have during the raising of one's children. All of these beliefs make children into "little idols" in one form or another. We hallow them and their achievements. Such idolatry, created by unresolved grief, not only blocks grieving, but blocks the opportunity to discover our children as adults. One of the tasks that parents need to accomplish if they are to pass through this transition well, is to de-idolize their children. The process needs to occur in the reverse direction as well. Our children need to de-idolize their parents. Both sides need to see each other's faults and strengths, and begin to relate to one another as human beings, if parenthood is to pass into friendship.

One of the things that helps parents avoid making idols out of their children is having other concerns and causes in their lives. Children are only a part of their parents' lives, not all of it. When parents start making the part into the whole, they have essentially created an idol. In the language of the social psychologist, Bernice Neugarten concludes that "to the extent that a woman has been able to build on her own individuality, major life transitions will be accomplished more smoothly."[13] This is why it is a wise piece of advice in parenting to save time and energy for other concerns. Have a career. Develop interests outside of the home. Invest yourselves in your marriage. This more balanced style of parenting actually helps the children. They benefit from being with parents who are alive and growing. They also benefit from not feeling so much pressure to be everything for their parents, to fulfill their unlived lives, to bolster their parents' shaky egos. Conversely, a more well-balanced parent finds the transition to the empty-nest easier.

Parents who have the most difficulty forming friendships with their adult children are often parents who have codependent traits. Codependency is a term derived from the twelve-step movement. It refers to the role of the spouse of the alcoholic, who is dependent on the drinking spouse remaining addicted. In this sense, the codependent person enables or unconsciously reinforces the partner's illness, because the codependent person needs to be needed. Often parents who cannot let go of their nearly adult children have similar traits, that is, their need to be needed blocks them from letting go of their children. When they feel they are not needed by their growing children, it creates deep feelings of anxiety and unworthiness. And then sometimes they subtly encourage their children not to become fully independent, so that at some level they are still needed as parents. Most of us have some codependent traits, it is part of what made us good parents when the children were younger. In the loss of family, God gives us an opportunity to look at ourselves, and grow out of our codependent traits.

Another related concept found in the codependency studies is the concept of boundaries. This refers to the psychological dividing line between what is my space, my problems, and my issues and yours. The term is derived from family systems theory. Families and individuals can have rigid or fluid boundaries. Some families are "enmeshed," that is, they have very weak boundaries between family members. In enmeshed families, boundaries and individual identities are not sharp, clear, nor mutually respected. Such families and the parents of such families often have a more difficult time allowing children to grow up, allowing children to be different, affirming their individuality, and claiming the autonomy of each family member. Such parents often find the loss of family to be frightening and respond with increasingly rigid defenses. Conversely, if we are to successfully travel through this passage, we must be willing to look at the boundary issues that will inevitably surface in our relationships with our adult children. We need to work hard at establishing and reestablishing and then respecting the boundaries between us and our adult children.[14]

If we work through the loss of family in a reasonable and timely fashion, great potential exists for new possibilities with these unique individuals we call children. If we can let go of our children as children, we create the possibility of relating to them as adults, even as friends. Few other losses in later life have this built-in potential. Not everyone is able to have an adult relationship with his or her children. There are many variables, some of which are out of our control. We are blessed if this kind of relationship occurs. Only then can we see them and ourselves as individuals. New life will emerge out of old, but only if we pass through the transition called the loss of family.

NEW POSSIBILITIES FOR CARING

Erik Erikson has written much on the seventh stage of the human life cycle, called Generativity. In this stage mature adults move toward investing themselves in caring for the next generation. Generativity is more than raising children, although it can include parenting. Generativity is most often associated with the empty-nest stage of life. Caring is the chief virtue to flower in mature adults during this period and it is expressed in their desire to invest themselves in people and causes larger than themselves.[15] Pastoral theologian Don S. Browning has suggested that this Generativity stage, if the crisis is resolved positively, is the zenith of the Christian journey.[16] This stage of life offers the clearest potential for the individual to become spiritually mature and in a sense is the goal toward which the Christian journey moves.

Like few other losses of the later years, the loss of family has great potential waiting for us on the other side of this transition. Many advantages and potentialities may be found in the empty-nest period of life, one of which is the opportunity to learn the virtue of care. We are invited to enter a new period, the generativity stage of life. But in order to care, to invest ourselves emotionally, we must let go of our emotional investments in the nuclear family—the children, the roles, lifestyle, and the meanings. Only as we process such losses, will we have the emotional energy to care in the stage of generativity awaiting us.

Chapter 5

The Loss of Parents

Honor your father and your mother, that your days may be long in the land which the Lord your God gives you.

Ex 20:12

All of us have parents. Our parents gave us life. They cared for us when we were helpless. They raised us. They molded and shaped our personalities for better or worse. When we were younger, we feared losing our parents. That was the most frightening nightmare we could imagine. That primal fear never really goes away. In the second half of life most of us will realize that fear. We will live to bury one, and probably both, of our parents.

THE AGING PARENT

It is no secret that the population of the United States is changing and becoming more "gray." The birthrate is declining in the United States, but more important for our purposes, the length of life is increasing. For a child born in 1989, the life expectancy is now approximately seventy-five years.[1] The combination of these factors means that the percentage of oldr people in the population, currently about 13 percent, is increasing and the trend is expected to continue well into the twenty-first century.[2] Most of us can relate to this larger cultural trend in very personal ways. Most of us have or will have parents that will live or are living well into their eighties or longer. The second half of life is inevitably filled with the issues and reactions to the aging and eventual death of our parents.

Sometimes the middle generation (ages thirty to sixty years) is called the "sandwich generation," because it is caught in the middle between the demands of aging parents and the responsibilities of growing children. This current generation of adult children is probably feeling the full impact of this squeeze more than any other generation prior to it. The declining birthrate, for example, means fewer adult children are available today to support and care for aging parents. In addition, the increased number of women who are employed outside of the home means that women, who are traditionally the caregivers, are less available to care for aging parents than in previous generations.[3] All this combines to make this generation of adult children feel more "caught" than most. Given the trends in the population, the prospects for the future do not appear to be much different.[4]

Another social trend that affects our relationships with our aging parents is the general mobility of our society. We are a very mobile people compared to other cultures and nations. It is not uncommon for parents and their adult children to live in distant towns or even states. In previous centuries, this was not the case. Sometimes two, three, or four generations of a family were all to be found living within a few miles of each other. This is still the pattern in many rural communities, but increasingly the norm is becoming more one of parents living in a separate residence from their children that may be in a distant town, city, or even state.[5] Telecommunications and affordable travel alleviate some of the effects of this distance. Most of us do talk with our parents regularly, but rarely do we see them on a daily basis.

The third cultural factor that impacts our personal relationships with our parents as they age is the cultural isolation of the elderly. As people enter "old age," whenever that is, they progressively move out of the mainstream of society into specialized facilities designed to meet their unique needs for socialization, health care, and the like. These facilities can include homes for the aged scattered throughout the community or whole villages devoted to serving the elderly. Eventually, when our parents' health declines, they may relocate again to a hospital, a hospice, or a nursing home. There is great convenience and wisdom in the trend toward specialized facilities for the elderly, although it is still only a trend. There are also several disadvantages. Chief among them is the isolation of the elderly from day-to-day contact and interaction with people of other generations. We and our parents are poorer for it.

All of these cultural trends combine to make it easy for us to avoid emotional involvement with our aging parents. They are not aging before our eyes, so to speak. We do not have to think about them very much. "Out of sight, out of mind," as the saying goes. The needs of the elderly, and in particular the needs of our parents, can easily get placed on the back burner of life. Some of this avoidance can be attributed to physical circumstances, but some of it is also an expression of our own denial mechanisms. Our denial is made easy by our culture's trend toward isolating the elderly. We can conveniently avoid them and our feelings about that impending loss.

Denial can be a two-way street. Many aging parents do not want to see themselves as aging. They can contribute to the collective denial by reassuring us when we phone periodically that "everything is fine here." Do you have a father who doesn't tell you when he goes in for surgery until after its over? Doesn't he say, "I didn't want to worry the kids?" Our parents don't want to be a burden or a bother to anyone, especially to their children. Most older people hate having to ask for help and they would certainly rather not be an object of pity. So, they too may avoid facing their own gradual aging and decline in physical well-being. And if we, their adult children, are also trying to avoid facing reality, the result can be a kind of collusion of denial. With this kind of collusion operating, it is easy to avoid dealing with our aging, and eventually dying, parents until it's too late to do much constructively.

AGING BRINGS CHANGES

As our parents age there are several subtle changes that occur in their psychology and in their interpersonal relationships with their adult children. These changes signal to us that we are losing them as parents, that they are declining in health, influence and energy. How we respond to these changes reflects our willingness to deal with our own feelings of loss and anxiety.

Considerable discussion in the literature on aging describes the increasing dependency that older people experience as they age after

sixty-five.[6] That dependency takes many forms. With health limitations, they need more assistance with the daily routines of shopping,
washing clothes, banking, etc. With a limited income, they may need
financial support from their adult children. And with decreasing energy, they must move to smaller quarters and perhaps to a health care
facility. The dependency is also psychological. Older people, particularly single people, are lonely. They need to socialize and they enjoy
talking about family and the past. If our single parent lives in isolation,
then he or she can become especially dependent on us.

"Every time I call Mama," says Yolanda, "she sounds so pathetic
and lonely. She could talk my ear off all day, if I let her. And it's
usually about old times or about the lousy job that her cleaning lady
does or how the mailman messed up her mail. She always ends the
conversation with, 'When are you coming to see me?'"

The corresponding concept that is frequently mentioned in the aging
literature is "role reversal." As our parents age, adult children experience a gradual reversal of the roles. Our parents become more dependent, more childlike, and we become more parentlike, supportive, and
nurturing of them. We begin to "parent our parents." We may start to
make decisions for them, give them advice, and in some cases literally
care for their physical needs, even as they cared for us when we were
infants in their arms.

Bruce, a middle-age child of an ailing parent, told me that his
mother would not take her medicine until he scolded her about its
importance. "At first," said Bruce, "it felt weird, scolding my mother.
She certainly gave me hell many times over the years, but then I began
to realize that it really wasn't a matter of who's the parent or child, it's
part of our family habit. That's how Mother knows I love her. That's
how she loved me. She wants me to scold her." So Bruce continued
scolding his mother quite regularly until the end, and when she did die
several years later, he scolded her for that too.

What these subtle changes in roles and psychology suggest is that
we begin to lose our parents as parents long before they actually die.
Our parents cease to function as parents as they decline in health and
energy. We begin to feel that they are not the tower of strength,
wisdom, and nurture that they have always been—or at least that is
how they seemed. We must be willing to allow our parents and our
relationship with our parents to change. Some adult children of aging

parents cannot do that. It's too frightening to let go of the image of their parents as strong, independent, available people. I would suggest that such people have made little idols of their parents or of a particular image of their parents. They cannot see their parents as individuals. They cannot allow their parents to change, because it shatters their rigid role definitions and subtle idolization.

It is difficult to watch one's parents age, to see their health deteriorate, to see them lose their love of life, to watch them narrow their lives and give up cherished goals. It may be difficult, also, to deal with their dependency and the subtle role reversal that occurs. It is difficult to see all of this happen in people whom we once so admired or feared or both. How will we respond to these changes? Can we deal with our own feelings of loss, so that we can accept the changes that are occurring and respond to our parents with kindness? Or will we hide behind our denial systems and avoid contact with them, continuing to force them not to be themselves so that we may keep our idolatrous images intact? As our parents age, we experience the first glimpses of their loss and respond accordingly.

As hard as it is to deal with our aging parents and their eventual deaths, there is a strong thrust in Western religious traditions toward caring for the elderly, and in particular, for one's parents. To some extent this tradition has been weakened by the forces of modern society, including secularism, mobility, and the isolation of age groups. Our ability to care for our aging parents is directly related to our willingness to face our own grief feelings about the emerging loss of our parents. Because we deny our own painful feelings of loss, we avoid, ignore, do not respect, and sometimes even ridicule our elderly parents. God wants us to care for the aging, but to do so, we must face our grief openly.

Did you ever notice a conditional clause in the fifth commandment, "Honor your father and mother. . . ?" The rest of the imperative reads, ". . . that your days may be long in the land the Lord God gives you." Honoring our parents will enable us to live long lives ourselves. That's a bit strange. Most people would think the opposite, that they might have less stress, and therefore live longer, if they ignore their aging parents. Yet, the commandment clearly implies that our ability to live long lives is dependent upon whether or not we honor our own parents. Catholic priest and professor of gerontology Leo Missinne has suggested that this commandment means that the more we are involved with our aged parents, the more we are preparing ourselves for our own aging.[7] We see are our future in our aging parents. We will cope better with our old age if we are involved with caring for our aging parents now.

THE SLOW DEATH

Death can come in various ways, but the long slow death is one of the most difficult to deal with. Modern medicine and hospitals being what they are, most of our parents will die in hospitals or nursing homes and most of them will have protracted dying processes. In contrast to the sudden death, the slow death allows us time to prepare ourselves for our parents' death. Yet, if the dying process becomes too long or too filled with suffering, we may reach the point where we start wanting our parents to die. Death can be a blessing for those who have suffered long. It can also come as a release for the adult child—a release from the long vigil.

The worst aspect of these kinds of deaths for the adult child is the emotional drain. Long terminal illnesses may involve several periods of hospitalization and eventually a longer stay in a nursing home and then, finally, death—or maybe even another brief recovery, followed by another round of illness. These are emotionally exhausting situations. It is as if we start and stop our own grief process again and again. Each time a crisis occurs, we begin to prepare ourselves emotionally to deal with the final loss of our parent. Then when our parent rallies, our grief is put on hold, only to be reactivated when the next crisis comes along. The emotional roller coaster of a chronic illness is taxing on all.[8]

Our parents, of course, would rather avoid such circumstances too. Most older people would rather die quickly than become prolonged financial and emotional burdens upon their families. Some families, therefore, try to decide in advance how they will handle slow deaths. Once our time comes, however, the situation becomes a different matter altogether. Now it is our mother in that hospital bed or our father in the nursing home. It is no longer a hypothetical example. We feel obligated to do everything possible to make Mom comfortable or give Dad every chance of recovery. It is not something that we can treat casually or intellectually. It's an emotional time.[9]

At the start of a parent's critical illness, it may not be clear to us what we're dealing with, whether this is the end or just the beginning of a long decline. We do not know if we are in for a sprint or a marathon. Initially, we drop what we are doing and rush to his or her side. But then the illness drags on and on, and at some point we must shift gears psychologically from a crisis mentality into a long-haul mentality. Somewhere in the middle of our current busy schedule, we must now find time for an ill parent, either in person or by phone or by semiregular trips. Inevitably our spouse and children get short-changed. Sometimes they come to resent our increased involvement, physically and emotionally, with our ill parent. Old family jealousies surface and we have even more stress to deal with—trying to care for the ill parent and trying to keep the spouse and children off our backs. All of this can and does affect how we handle the slow death of an aging parent. Little wonder that when Mom or Dad does pass on, we may feel a sense of relief—for them and for ourselves.

When Jean returned from burying her ninety-two-year-old mother, she was more relieved than sorrowful. "Mother had been ill so long," she said, "and suffered so long. I think that she wanted to go at the end. She just waved off people. She wouldn't take her pills or cooperate with the nurses. I think she wanted to die at that point—and who can blame her?" Because of this situation, Jean's grieving process was different. There was more relief in her grief, more of a mixture of gratitude and sorrow. Several weeks after her mother's death, she said, "It's not as bad as I thought it would be. I thought I would be devastated when Mom died, but it's manageable. Oh, sure, I miss her, but it's not the way I felt after Dad's sudden death. Dad's death was horrible. Mom's death is—OK." Most of us who have suffered through and with our parents' dying can empathize with Jean's mixture of feelings. The loss of a parent after a long, slow dying is an ambivalent experience and therefore an ambivalent grief.

Middle-aged adults of the "sandwich generation" have responsibilities on both ends of life. Besides the ill or aging parent, they also have busy work schedules, family obligations, and household duties that can't wait. Amidst all of this, there is little time to grieve. It is easy for busy adult children to ignore their own grief for their dying or deceased parent. It is easy just to repress it or deny it or drown it in activity. It doesn't seem as important as all the pressing obligations of career and family.

THE IGNORED GRIEF

The loss of parents is difficult for many adults because its grief is largely ignored and undervalued in our society. The grief that adults feel when their parent(s) die is a secret grief. It is the hidden pain that millions of adults carry around with them year after year. Edward Myers in his book, *When Parents Die* expresses this same point of view when he writes:

> In fact, our entire culture has more or less ignored what adults experience following the death of their parents. Yet, five per-cent of the United States population loses a parent within a given year. Given our current population, that means that 11,650,000 Americans lose a parent annually. Loss of a parent is the single most common form of bereavement in this coun-try. . . . [Yet] the unstated message is that when a parent is middle-aged or elderly, the death is somehow less of a loss than other losses. The message is that grief for a dead parent isn't entirely appropriate.[10]

We live in an age when there is a virtual epidemic of unresolved grief in our society. Millions upon millions of people carry the pain of a loss with them, just below the surface of their psyches. One of the largest, if not the largest, category of losses that remain un-healed is that of a death of a parent.

There are probably several reasons why this particular loss gets downgraded in the culture. Most people think, for example, that when a parent dies, it was expected or should have been expected. "After all, every parent will die someday." That is a normal part of life. People should expect it and therefore, by implication, should not be as upset emotionally. Second, most parents die in old age after long lives. Therefore, the assumption is that the survivors should not grieve as intensely as they might if the parent had died during their youth. "After all they had their life." Third, when a parent dies, much of the focus of the supportive community is on the grieving spouse, not on the grieving adult child. When John's father died, he noted, "The first question out of people's mouths was, 'How is your mom doing?' The first question was rarely, if ever, 'How are you doing?'" The assumption is made that an adult son's or daughter's grief should not be as intense as a spouse's. That may or may not be true. Much depends on circumstances. They are different losses and most likely different griefs. In many people's minds, however, the surviving child is a grown-up, a responsible middle-generation adult. He or she doesn't need our sympathy and support the way the lonely spouse does. Thus, the grief of the adult child gets ignored.

The result of this observation, if true, is that it is diificult to grieve openly for our parents. We tend to bottle up the emotions faster than we might otherwise. We tend to think that we should get over it sooner and get back to work, back to our many responsibilities. There are few social supports for the mourning for our aged parents. So we don't grieve. And if our parent died an agonizing death, then we are all the more relieved than grieved. It is hard to appreciate our pain, when our mind keeps telling us how much better off he or she is.

GUILT IN GRIEF

Compared to other losses and other griefs, the grief we feel for our deceased parent(s) seems unusually permeated with guilt feelings. Guilt is a normal component of grieving, but it seems especially prevalent in the mourning we experience after a parent's death.

Prior to the 1978 national conference on "You and Your Aging Parent," approximately one hundred unstructured interviews were conducted with people involved in all dimensions of the issue. Ira S. Hirschfield and Helen Dennis report: "For the adult child, the most dominant and pervasive issue regarding intergenerational relationships is the subject of guilt."[11] People feel obligated to their parents—a sense of responsibility. They want "to do right by them," especially during their last years or days of life. Guilt is a theme as one's parent ages, but it is also the dominant theme in the bereavement of the adult child. After Mom or Dad dies, we need some reassurance that we did all we could, that there are no loose ends, that our obligations were fulfilled. Our successful adjustment to the loss of a parent must involve the resolution of our guilt feelings.

In reference to our parents, most of us feel a generalized guilt left over from our childhood. We all have long histories, filled with pleasant and painful memories. Most of us have numerous events or issues that we feel guilt about with our parents—some things we did not perform well, some words we shouldn't have said, some obligations we forgot about. Usually these are events that have long since been forgotten by our parents—but not by us. Just below the surfaces of our adult facades, there is still a little girl or a little boy that wants Daddy's recognition or Mommy's embrace more than anything else in all the world. And in the mind of that little girl or little boy, we still may feel that we have never quite earned either the recognition or the embrace. This kind of generalized guilt is almost universal with parents and their adult children. It is there in our grieving.

Sometimes the guilt in our grief is related to the unexpressed anger or resentments we feel toward our parents. Physician Smiley Blanton, writing about the middle-aged adult, says:

> We must always keep in mind the psychiatric truth that where our parents are concerned we have an ambivalent attitude: we love them, but we also resent them . . . The memory of them still exists in us, below the conscious level, and the corresponding resentments exist too.[12]

We all feel some disappointment in our parents. It's an inevitable part of growing up. Some people work throught this disappointment before their parents die. Others who do not carry their resentment into their bereavement. It is hard to be angry with the deceased when we're supposed to feel sorrowful. "I'm angry, but I can't be angry. I feel guilty that I feel angry at these 'wonderful' people to whom I should be eternally grateful." Do you hear the guilt in the anger?

Another part of the guilt that we might feel in relation to our parents' death may have to do with particular decisions we had to make for Mom or Dad involving their living arrangements or medical care. If we had to place Mom in a nursing home against her wishes, then that can bother us. Or if we decided to let Dad live alone after Mom died, instead to taking him into our home, we may feel guilty about that. Or if we were not able to be present at the moment of death, then that may bother us. Or if we were not as supportive or as thoughtful as we felt we should have been (or as much as a sibling was), then that may bother us too.[13] All of these real or perceived "sins" may trouble us and become the particulars of our guilt.

In the process of losing our parents, it is almost impossible to avoid having to make difficult medical, legal, and financial decisions regarding our parents' welfare. Here is where we really earn our keep as sons or daughters. There are no easy decisions, and if this is our last parent and if we are also the only child available, then the burden of these decisions falls squarely on our shoulders. In particular, the medical decisions and the question of "heroic measures" lingers in the back of our minds. Most of us are laypersons when it comes to the high-tech world of modern medicine and hospital care. We can be easily overwhelmed and confused by conflicting medical terms, procedures, and even the different types of doctors. How far should we go in trying to prolong a parent's life? How far would Mom or Dad want us to go? When is there no chance for a full recovery, or even a partial recovery? When do we "pull the plug?" And who makes that decision?[14]

Working with guilt feelings seems to be a process of sorting through the events, scenes and conversations that bother us most. Part of our grief work is to talk through all of the factors and situations. The troublesome events may be recent or those of many years earlier. Sometimes we have to go over them again and again, so as to clear our minds. We have to try to decide if we did the right thing or the not-so-right thing. The only solution for legitimate guilt is a full acceptance of God's forgiveness. Some of the guilt feelings associated with bereavement are not so legitimate though, and we must wrestle more with forgiving ourselves.

Tony tortured himself for years about his mother's death. "It was handled all wrong," he thought. "I wasn't there when she died, as she requested. You know she asked me to do that, on the phone about a week before she died. She said, 'Honey, when the time comes, you be here. Will you?' I assured her that I would be there. She had always counted on me since Dad died. She was really scared of dying alone."

Unfortunately, Tony's mother did die alone in the middle of the night. Tony couldn't get there fast enough. Now he can't forgive himself. Intellectually, he knows that he couldn't have gotten there, but emotionally he can't let go of it. It hurts too much. The image of his mother dying alone haunts him. "After all that Mother did for me, that was the least I could have done for her," he mourned, "but I couldn't come through."

I remember the day that Tony began to get some relief from this guilt. It came during a dramatic role play that he and a woman therapist were engaged in. In acting out an imaginary conversation between Tony and his mother, the therapist kept saying "I forgive you. . . . I forgive you. . . . I forgive you." I must have counted twenty times that this phrase was said, and each time the words cut deeper and deeper into Tony's soul. He had never really let those words in so deep before. Up to now he had known about forgiveness, but had not experienced it. Tony's tears flowed long and hard. It was a different kind of grief now, a grieving for his failure, for his lost ideal, for his sins. It made possible the beginning of self-forgiveness.

BAGGAGE FROM THE PAST

We have a tendency to idealize our parents just by virtue of their being our parents. We all begin life as very dependent creatures called children. During those years we perceive our parents to be like gods. That is how it appears from the vantage point of a three-year-old. Mother and Father appear to be all-powerful, ever-present, and all-knowing. A part of the normal developmental process is a growing out of this kind of primitive dependency or parental idolatry. In time we come to see our parents as humans. Like us they are prone to mistakes; like us, they cannot be everywhere at once; and like us, they are not perfect. Yet, not everyone comes to this kind of mature perspective on his or her parents. Some people still make Mom or Dad into little gods, giving them unusual powers to determine their values and their self-worth. In grief, the tendency to idolize is even stronger, fueled as it is by a mistaken desire to honor their memory.

Joan's relationship with her father had always been a rocky one. As a child, the only girl, she wanted her father's attention, but could never seem to get it no matter how hard she tried. He was a critical and demanding father who gave little praise but plenty of advice. During her adolescent years she rebelled often and did some pretty foolish things, all designed in one way or another to attract his attention. Her father just ignored her even more. He seemed to be more interested in her brothers and their assorted accomplishments than in Joan's antics. Joan grew into adulthood, feeling that she was never going to be good enough.

Over the years, Joan's father mellowed a great deal and Joan grew up, married, and had a family. Dad seemed to converse more with her as he got older. He wasn't so crusty and aloof. He seemed to take genuine delight in Joan's children, who in turn loved going to visit their grandpa. Only through her own children did Joan feel any partial approval by her father. Yet, it was an ambivalent feeling for Joan to see her father bestowing more affection on her children than she felt she ever received from him herself.

Following her father's untimely death, all of these old issues surfaced in her grief. Joan's bereavement was permeated by depression. She had a sickening sense that it was now too late to earn his respect, too late to rescue her self-esteem. To make matters worse, she had failed him again. Her mom reported that two days before he died, he was complaining that Joan did not bring the grandchildren by to see him. Joan can see the frown on his face as clear as day. Even from his grave, he was disapproving of her. Now in her grief she longed for his love all the more. Through her tears, she would say, "If only he was still here, even for a day, perhaps he would love me. Perhaps we would have that conversation that I always wanted to have." Yet in her calm moments, she knew so well that words had always been difficult between them. Despair dominated her grieving. It seemed that there was no chance for her now, no hope. All of her self-acceptance was buried with him. From her perspective, she was left with nothing but her inadequacies.

Joan had great trouble with her grief work. On one hand she idolized her father more in her sorrow than she had done in real life. Daddy became all-powerful in death. His approval alone mattered—but now there was no hope. She would never earn his respect now. She was condemned to live out her days without full acceptance.

Obviously Joan had much baggage left over from the past that contaminated her grief process. She never experienced much healing until she recognized all of this baggage and began to wrestle with the whole of her relationship with her father. In the terminology of this book, she "idolized" her father. Her operational theology read, "I will be saved only when Father approves of me" and she carried this belief right into her bereavement. In fact, grieving only intensified the feelings. Ultimately for Joan, salvation was not to be found in worshipping the dead, but in taking back her own power and then in rooting her worth in a God whose love transcends the losses and idols of this world.

CAN'T GO HOME AGAIN

Another theme experienced by many in the loss of their parents is the awareness that they have lost more than these two individuals. They have lost the parents of yesterday, the parents of their childhood and youth.

In grieving over a parent's death, there is tendency to review all of the memories of childhood. John, for example, says that when his father died, he remembered the times they went fishing together when he was a kid. "All through the funeral," John related, "I kept thinking of one fishing trip after another. They were good memories, tender memories, but I hadn't thought of most of them in years." In grieving for our parents, we remember the full scope of our history with them.

Yes, we know that we lost our childhood years ago when we grew up and left home. It seemed OK then. We were going on to something else. But now when our parents die, we feel as if we are losing our childhood all over again. Maybe we are losing our history. Our parents are the keepers of the hundred and one funny stories about our child-hood. They know all of our past.[15] They know who we were and how we have become what we are. We grieve for both our parents and our childhood.

When my own father lay dying in a hospital, each of us had time to make our peace with him. That was one of the few advantages of his prolonged battle with death. I remember my last words to him so well. Dad had drifted off into a coma a couple days earlier, so most of my last time with him was just me sitting hold his hand, talking to him here and there. The time had come for me to leave. I knew very well this might be my last time to see him alive. The words just came tumbling out, "Good-bye, Daddy. I love you." I was a little bit sur-prised at them myself. I hadn't called him "Daddy" in probably thirty years, but it seemed right. It was as though I was saying good-bye not just to the "dad" of today, but to the "daddy" of yesterday too. "Good-bye, Daddy."

People have a strange intangible feeling about their parents and their home. No matter how old we get, we think that we can always go home again. It was the poet Robert Frost who defined home as that place where if you go there, they have to take you in. Middle-age adults really don't go home much, but it's nice to know that it is there.

"Sometimes when I am sick with a cold," says Holly, "but I can't stop to rest—kids must get to practice, the laundry is piling up—I say to myself, 'I'm going home to Mom. She will make me a big bowl of homemade soup,'" Holly fantasizes, "and I'll curl up on the couch with a good book, watch a little TV, and Mom and I will talk until 2 a.m." Part of us, like Holly, thinks that we can always go home again, even if we never do. When our parents die, that fantasy is shattered. We can't go home again.

The process of working through our parents' will, estate, and personal possessions evokes similar kinds of feelings. The process of dissolving the family home carries with it many of these same feelings of the loss. Have you had the experience of sitting down with your siblings and dividing up the possessions of your parents' home? It is an unpleasant task, one that many of us would just as soon avoid. It can be very sad. Each possession or memento is a part not just of their lives, but of our life as well. We have memories and feelings about our parents' possessions. We have not just lost them, our beloved parents, but we have lost a part of ourselves—our past, our childhood, our home.

NEW IDENTITY, NEW LIFE STAGE

All losses have an eschatological dimension to them. All losses make us aware of the shortness of time. The death of one's parent(s) seems to accent this awareness in a special way. We, the adult children, become more aware that the older generation has passed on and that now our generation rises to the position of leadership. This awareness changes family roles and identities.

When Jim's father died, he reported, "I was aware of how I became the eldest man in the family. There was no one else to look up to. My younger sister used to call Dad a lot, but now she calls me. Dad's death made a difference in my role. I wasn't sure I was ready for it. There is a part of me that doesn't want to be head of this family. I don't want the responsibility. I'm not that old." The death of a parent inevitably brings on these kinds of changes in family dynamics and interactions. In a sense dying is a family affair.

When Cloyce's father died, she was approaching a midlife crisis. He was a well-known minister in the New York City area, a popular speaker, and an influential and strong personality. He died unexpectedly of a heart attack after church one day. There were hundreds at his funeral. As the oldest child of four, Cloyce participated in the funeral service, saying some things on behalf of the family. That was when it really hit her that she had to do it. She had wanted to be a minister, but in those days women just didn't become ministers, and she kept waiting for one of the boys to follow in Dad's footsteps. They never did, and meanwhile she did everything but preach in her local church. There was something about his death that crystallized her own call. She knew that it was now or never. The following week she enrolled in the seminary. Her only regret was that her father couldn't have been there to officially "lay on the hands" in her ordination ceremony three years later. He would have been proud.

Something about the death of one's parents seems to make us aware of this "now or never" dimension to life. And when the loss of our parents corresponds to our own midlife crisis, the sense of time is heightened even more.[16] Now we are the next generation. The torch has been passed. Our role has changed. We have a new identity and a new opportunity for growth. We may pick up the torch or not, as we wish. But regardless, the torch has been passed. The death or our parents has a way of calling us to be what we are meant to be.

The world is a different place after our parents die. On the one hand the world seems emptier now, stripped of illusions and comforts, more alone in a deep existential way. On the other hand, when our parents die, we seem to come of age. We pass into a new stage in life's journey, a time of generativity, a time of "filial maturity," a time of fulfillment. We now take our place "center stage." We take up the artist's brushes and for better or worse leave our mark on life's canvas. This new life stage can be the most productive and creative of our life cycle. But it will be so only if we are able to say "goodbye" to our parents and not cling to them in varying degrees of idolization. The living God bids us to grieve. For only in grief will we again find new life.

Chapter 6

The Loss of Work

> . . . and they burned incense to other gods, and worshiped the works of their own hands.

> Jer 1:16

Most all of us work throughout the adult years, both inside and outside the home. Most of us invest ourselves in our jobs. We take pride in our jobs, because they reflect on us and give our lives meaning. In our adult years, we tend to define ourselves by our work. Some of us even have something more than a job. We have a lifelong investment in a particular line of work or area of activity. We have a career.

So it is, then, that one of the major losses in the later years is the loss of work. Sooner of later, each of us will give up, voluntarily or involuntarily, our life's work. This loss may come abruptly, such as at retirement, or it may come gradually as we reduce our duties with our increasing age. Eventually, we must give up our work and all the feelings of worthiness, identity, and productivity that go with it.

THE CHANGING FACE OF RETIREMENT

"Retirement" in its present-day form is really an invention of the twentieth century. During most of the history of Western civilization and certainly in other cultures today, people did not retire in the modern sense of the word. There was no set period of leisure at the end of life that one was entitled to as a reward for years of labor. Most humans continued to work every day of their lives and gave up work only as their decreasing energy led them to. As they aged and could not carry the expected workload, they moved into the roles of teacher, master craftsman, or counselor to the younger workers. A person was never completely uninvolved in his or her craft, business, or family farm. There was always work to be done. "Retirement," if anything, meant a much smaller period of time, usually when one was totally disabled or unable to work. In those days, nobody wanted to be retired.

The nature of retirement did not change in isolation. Two other social changes helped make possible the modern retirement we now enjoy. One of the factors was the financing of retirement. The Social Security program was the first step in that direction. It was the first large-scale source of retirement income outside of earned wages. Even more important, the Social Security program changed people's expectations. Now retirement was seen more as a time to be enjoyed. For that kind of retirement, however, money was needed. More and more people began creating pension funds, annuities, and savings. Others began to demand that these benefits be built into the contractual agreements between employees and employers.

Second, advances in health care have made retirement more enjoyable, more of a period of leisure instead of a brief period forced on us by declining health. It is now possible to retire in good health and spend many years enjoying life before encountering severe health limitations. The life expectancy of Americans has steadily increased throughout this century. Without these advances in affordability and in health care, retirement would not be possible as it is currently constituted.

When should one retire? The wisdom on this subject has changed over the years. Through the mid-part of this century, the mandatory retirement age of sixty-five was accepted and generally enforced. Yet, there has always been a great debate about the values of compulsory retirement.[1] Many prefer retirement to be a fixed point, in which it could be anticipated and planned for and in which people would be "required" to let go of their work. Others resent having to give up work while they still have many good years left.

The old adage that "retirement brings early death" fed into this debate on the necessity of a fixed retirement age. There seemed to be many stories of high-strung workaholics who retired abruptly and dropped dead within two weeks. When this adage was put under the scrutiny of research, however, it did not hold up.[2] The data now suggest that there is no link between retirement per se and early death. In fact, the opposite relationship may well be true: retirement prolongs life in most cases. The health of older citizens has generally improved so much in recent decades that now the "health argument" is used as a reason for extending the mandatory retirement age to seventy.

Currently, there is great flexibility in this nation on the subject of when to retire. Many professions, companies, and unions are approaching the subject with an open mind. They are trying to look at the "abilities and capabilities" of the individual instead of any fixed age. There are more and more early retirements. In 1980, for example, the majority of eligible retirees, retired before the age of sixty-five.[3] Many of these people took retirement at age sixty-two, which is now permissible in the Social Security system. Some executives are given incentives to retire earlier than that to make room for a new management team. Police officers and firefighters can retire after twenty years of service and some professional athletes retire at age thirty-five when their bodies cannot keep up with the pace. At the other end of the scale, there are more people who choose to continue working long after age sixty-five. One estimate is that 20 percent to 30 percent of retirees continue to work on a part-time basis.[4]

These changes in the face of retirement seem to be largely welcomed and appear to be healthy changes.[5] There is such diversity among people in the later years that it seems wise to provide more options for people regarding retirement. The implication of all this for our discussion about loss of work is that the loss of work is no longer as much of a fixed event as it used to be. The loss of work is experienced by more and more people as a gradual process.

RETIREMENT AND THE MEANING OF WORK

What is clear from much of the research on retirement is that how one deals with retirement depends in large measure on the meaning that work has for that person prior to retirement. This observation should sound familiar. In our earlier discussion of grief dynamics, we noted that the strength of a person's sorrow depends on the meaning that he or she gives to the lost object. The issue is not just the strength of the meaning, however, but the varieties of meanings and unique functions that working performs in our lives. What is clear is that work carries several important meanings in our lives. We need to understand these meanings if we are to understand the nature of the loss of work.

Robert Havighurst has been associated with the study of work and retirement for three decades. His book, *The Meaning of Work and Retirement,* co-authored with Eugene A. Friedmann, is a classic in this field.[6] The studies therein have been repeated in many other times and places. The conclusions have largely stood the test of time, although they have been expanded with each new study. The central conclusion of Havighurst's research is that a link exists between the significance a person attaches to work and that person's adjustment to retirement.

After studying various occupational groups for many years, Havighurst currently suggests that there are six broad "social psychological meanings of work."[7] These extend beyond the obvious purpose of work which is to provide income. The six larger meanings are:

1. Work is the basis for our sense of worth or self-respect. We feel good about ourselves when we work.
2. Work is a locus of social participation. We make friends and maintain friendships through our jobs.
3. Work is a source of prestige. We get recognition through the quality of our work.
4. Work includes new experiences, a chance to be creative and to achieve. Work is a means of self-expression.
5. Work is a chance to serve others. This meaning is more associated with service-oriented work.
6. Work is a way of passing time. Work is a way of avoiding boredom.

These various purposes of work vary according to the occupational group being studied. People from all occupational groups affirm that work is a source of friends, a way of passing time and a means of gaining self-respect. Some occupational groups emphasize "service to others" more than other groups, and the "new experiences" meaning is found only among people in the arts or similar creative professions. All occupations, however, do carry some, if not all, of these extra-economic meanings. Work encompasses much more than a source of income. Therefore, the loss of work is important too.

Over the years Havighurst and other researchers[8] have demonstrated a strong link between retirement adjustment and the significance of work. They found that the people who viewed work only as a way to earn money and had few extra economic meanings attached to their work actually preferred to retire. Such people were usually the un-skilled or semiskilled workers who are largely unsatisfied in their work, and/or people who worked for a large employer.[9] Professional people, self-employed individuals, and highly satisfied workers usually found retirement much more difficult, and often resisted giving up their work identity in retirement.[10] In other words, if our work is nothing more than a job, then we can easily relinquish it. But retire-ment is much more difficult if our work is also our source of self-worth, our main source of social contacts, and our primary identity. Work means more to us, quantitatively and qualitatively. It becomes a complex loss, embedded with many sublosses.

This understanding of the role of meaning in loss adjustment fits with our understanding of grief and bereavement. We have learned that if the lost object or lost person means more to us, then we will experi-ence it as a greater loss and will grieve accordingly. If we assigned few meanings to that which is lost, then we will grieve lightly and easily, because our essential meanings are rooted elsewhere. The issue be-comes then: How central is work to our lives? How many extra mean-ings do we attach to our work? Does our job carry this extra baggage for us? If so, then when we lose work, in part or totally, we are losing more than a mere job. We are losing self-esteem, self-definition, a source of friends, and so on. From this perspective, we can readily see that the loss of work can be a significant loss in the life cycle that involves several powerful sublosses.

Meanings reflect human needs. Work provides a purpose to ful-fill important and necessary needs. Every human being needs to have friends, self-respect, a clear and stable identity, and so on. The problem of adjusting to retirement might then be understood as how to attain this need fulfillment in ways not associated with work. The needs are legitimate, and if they are not fulfilled in some way, a person's mental health will suffer in retirement. "The problem of retirement," writes Havighurst in the 1954 study, "is to secure the extra-economic values that work brings and to secure them through play or leisure-time activities. . . ."[11] In other words, if we are to adjust well to retirement, we must learn how to get self-respect and how to make and keep friends through leisure activities rather than exclusively through the workplace. Havighurst has argued that leisure is capable of fulfilling all of these needs if we correctly understand the nature of leisure and learn the "arts of leisure." Furthermore, he suggests that our society will continue to become more leisure oriented, as we live longer and as we become more affluent as a nation. Therefore, for Havighurst and others, the problem of retirement is a problem of leisure.[12]

THE LOSS OF STATUS

A recurrent theme with retired persons is the loss of status or power that they feel is associated with their loss of work. Admittedly, this theme is more reflective of persons who had some status or power in their jobs. Executives, professionals, and owners of businesses seem to feel this loss most keenly. This is not an issue for employees with little job status or authority.

Vern was a merchant all of his life. He learned the trade from his European father, although not the specific business. Vern started a small grocery store when he was a young man and grew up with it and through it. The store, "Vern's Market," was on the corner of Main and Elm, a landmark in this midwestern town. The store provided him with a good but modest income over the years. His four children were raised in the store, helping out on Saturdays, stocking shelves, sweeping floors. Sometimes he paid them a small wage. Sometimes it was just expected. Over the years Vern's store grew with the town. He expanded several times, buying two adjacent buildings, adding hardware lines, home products, and various services. In his later years, the store was more than he could handle. He gradually turned it over to his youngest son, who was the only child of the four who showed much interest in the place. Vern couldn't do the work anymore, but he still liked to call the shots from the back room.

Retirement was never discussed in Vern's family as such. It happened gradually. Vern had to give up the early morning trips to the produce mart, and Johnny began to do those tasks. As Vern's activities decreased, Johnny assumed a greater and greater role in the daily management of the store. It was difficult for Vern to see Johnny in his former role, especially when he did things differently from Vern.

Johnny had some new ideas that he wanted to try out, but was reluctant to go against father's wishes. Johnny didn't feel free to implement his ideas, because Dad was still "in charge"—sort of. Vern couldn't stay out of the store, but neither could he keep up with the demands. The conflicts increased, and at one point Johnny threatened to quit: "Either you let me run the store or you run it yourself, Dad. You can't have it both ways. It's time for you to let go of it." That seemed to help Vern see the issue more clearly. Johnny was right. Vern didn't want the hard work of the store, but he did like having the reins of power. It was the power that was most difficult to relinquish.

About this time, I asked Vern what he missed most about work. Vern replied "Not the work . . . too hard now, too difficult! You have to get up so early in the morning, and the 'fussy customers.' No, I don't miss that.

"I miss being the boss though. I like making my own decisions. I like the fact that everyone in town knows me.

"It was hard for me to let Johnny take over. He's a good boy, but I was so afraid he was going to ruin everything I have built up. It was real hard to watch him do it his way."

Vern did have a hard time giving up the power associated with his work, as modest as it was. About a year after this interview, however, he and his wife went on a six-month tour of the nation in a motor home. It was something that he always had wanted to do, but in retailing "you don't get many vacations." It was a delightful experience—the vacation that he never had. It also helped to separate him emotionally from his work. When he got back, Johnny was finally and really in charge.

How people adjust to retirement depends on what they are losing. If their job had status, then they lose status. Yet responsibility can be a burden as well as a privilege, as any merchant like Vern could tell us. Some retirees, when they really stop and think about it, are just as glad to get out from under the burden of power. Usually what they miss most is the trappings of power. They miss the status, the money, the prestige, the ability to order people around and get what they want when they want it.

Unfortunately, few rituals formalize and facilitate retirement or the transfer of power. Retirement parties come closest. Installation ceremonies also try to facilitate transfers of power. Facilitating the loss of work can sometimes be helped by finding ways to help retirees maintain a sense of status, even in retirement. Titles such as Professor Emeritus help those who have retired to see themselves as still valuable. A good ritual would both comfort the participants and facilitate their grieving.

LOSS OF FRIENDS

Most people find that their work is a place for making friends. Its degree of importance will vary from person to person. Some people make lifelong friends in and through their work. Others form work-only friendships. Either way, work friendships can be an important part of our social network and support system.

There is something very profound about the nature of work being communal. Work forces humans to cooperate. Several anthropologists, notably Richard Leakey, believe that the key to the success of human evolution is cooperation, not competition.[13] It wasn't that humans were more competitive or more aggressive than other species, but that humans were more cooperative than other species. Cooperation has led to our dominance as a species. Work requires that humans cooperate. Work throws people together in a common task, sometimes in common suffering, and thereby creates friendship. Often what we miss most in the loss of work is the daily contact with friends, the espirit de corps, and the genuine joy in a job well done.

Vivian is a seventy-one-year-old retired schoolteacher. She began her career in midlife, after her husband died an early death in an auto accident. She needed a job in those days to finish raising her two girls. She worked as an elementary schoolteacher, mostly in the same school, for over twenty-five years. She retired late, at age seventy, according to the new flexible retirement rules adopted by the school district. The last few years of her career, she was made a Master Teacher and spent a portion of her day coaching the younger teachers (actually they were all younger than she) in the art of teaching. In retirement she lived alone, not too far from the school where she worked for so long.

"The thing I miss most about my work," she remarked once, "is the children. I miss the children. I loved having children around me. I loved helping them, seeing them master a concept or paint a picture or sound out words for the first time. They were like a big family to me, and every year I got a new bunch. Some of them still keep in touch with me, you know. . . . I cannot take it like I used to, though. They wear me out more now. I miss the children, but I am also glad not to have them around all the time.

"I miss the school and my fellow teachers," she continued. "Teaching really became my social life during those years after Willard died. I socialized with my fellow teachers. Some of them became my best friends; in fact, they still see me occasionally and send me cards on my birthday and all. . . . It was hard adjusting to living without friends at first. I do not think that I have done it very well. I get lonely still and sometimes I just go for a walk, down past the school."

If our work is the main source of friendships over the years, then we are in for a difficult transition to retirement. We may want to find some way to stay involved marginally with our career, even if just for the social contacts. Other retirees may need to find new sources of friendship. There are many sources of friendship besides work—service clubs, neighborhoods, churches, interest groups, and so on, but they all must be pursued.

What many people discover in retirement is that their work was a built-in source of friends. Friendship was automatic, and so they didn't have to work at it. After they retire, however, the friendship isn't so automatic. They have to be more intentional about friendship. They have to work at it. It won't happen otherwise. They have to make it happen. This shift in one's expectations about friends and friendships is subtle but very important. Some retirees do not make this shift and just sit at home wondering why they are lonely.

The nice thing about being intentional about friendship is that we can choose *not* to socialize too. When we worked for a living, we were thrown together with people whether we wished to be or not. There were probably a few people that we did not want to socialize with, but were expected to. To some extent we had to socialize in the workplace. In retirement, however, we have the freedom not to socialize and to be more selective about our friends. Friendship is now intentional, something we have to choose. This is both pleasant and difficult.

The loss of friendship is one of the dimensions of the loss of work that can be difficult for many people. It involves a restructuring of where and how one socializes. It involves learning to work at making friends perhaps more than one had to in the past. Yet, making and maintaining friendships in old age is very important. It is one of the factors that is positively correlated with good mental and physical health. So, adjusting well to the loss of work must include learning to be intentional about friendship.

RETIREMENT AND THE IDOLIZATION OF WORK

When we lose work, either totally or partially, we go through an adjustment process that can resemble grief. So many variables influence the character of this process that it is hard to describe a uniform process for everyone. Much depends on the meanings that we have attached to our work and on how much preparation, emotionally and financially, we have done for retirement. Nevertheless, it is not uncommon to have feelings of loss, confusion, and meaninglessness during the first few months after retirement. In such situations, it is important to try to identify what exactly we are grieving. Are we grieving the loss of work? the loss of status? the loss of friends? or the loss of income? We can be grieving any and all of these things.

In time most people adjust to retirement. They learn to find new activities. They learn to find new sources of friends and new purposes. They learn to live with reduced income. But what if they do not adjust? What about the person who can't seem to let go of work and all that it has meant to him or her?

Terry was a career police officer. He had wanted nothing else when he was a kid. After high school he went directly to a two-year college and then applied for admission to the police academy. As an officer, he worked hard. He enjoyed his work. It was everything that he ever wanted a job to be. He made wonderful friendships with his fellow officers. "There is nothing like being under fire together to bring people close," he would say. Terry played on the police soft-ball team after hours. He worked out with weights during break times. He enjoyed every aspect of his career—the image, the social-izing, the work.

Terry was forty-two years old when his car crashed while chasing another vehicle. He was seriously injured and was hospitalized for several months. His injury involved the spinal cord and resulted in only partial use of his legs. This was a major trauma for Terry and his wife, but the police force was supportive and Terry's faith was strong. He was convinced that he could repair the damage with physical therapy and weight training. He'd be back on the active duty roster in no time. Well, Terry did work hard, but progress did not come after a year nor even after two years. Finally, he was forced to apply for disability retirement. Terry's police career was over.

Retirement was not welcomed. Terry had largely denied this possibility during his struggle for recovery. He was so convinced that he could recover. Once he was declared disabled, it seemed to snap his will to fight and he gave up. He spent most of the first several months just sitting watching television. Terry did receive some disability income, but it was much less than his full salary. This added insult to injury. Now Terry's wife had to take a job. Given Terry's state of mind, she was not entirely confident in his ability to handle the children. So she arranged her work schedule so that she would be finished about the time that the children came home from school. Terry had gone into a deep depression. Yet, he didn't want any help, even from the department's psychiatrist. It was hard for Terry to identify his feelings, much less talk them through. It was just not part of the image.

After a while, Terry began to visit the police station in the mornings. He would just hang around the coffee pot for several hours. He would time his visits so that he would have coffee with the morning shift. Most of his former colleagues did not mind Terry hanging around the station. He could be useful at times. So this pattern continued for almost another year. Terry enjoyed the station time. It helped him to feel as though he was still a police officer.

In time, however, a new commander arrived at the station, and he was a person who liked to run things by the book. He confronted Terry one day, ordering him not to come by the station anymore. "Listen, Terry, this is against regulations—you hanging around here. You are not an officer. Face it. You've got to get that through your head. It's time you go."

Terry resented those words. Angry, he stormed out of the station. He brooded about it for weeks, threatening "to sue the s.o.b." Yet the confrontation did force things into the open and as a result Terry sought professional help.

Terry's dynamics were a classic case of idolatry. His job was everything to him. More than a means of earning a living, it was also his identity. He loved the uniform, the muscles, the force, the macho image—all of it! Police work was his life. Nothing else mattered as much. Without it, as he was now, he felt useless, like "a nobody." "If only this accident hadn't happened," he would say, "if only the doctors had fixed me up better, if only the stupid police regulations allowed me to work some, then I would be happy." According to Terry, happiness could be found only in going backward, not forward.

Terry got some help for himself and his idolatry. The secret of Terry's recovery was not at all mysterious. Basically, Terry needed to grieve. He needed to identify and express his painful feelings of loss, including sorrow, anger, guilt, and depression. He needed to refashion his belief system to find meaning for himself in something apart from work. For Terry, a part of his recovery was found in returning to an active faith in his church. He needed to root himself "in something beyond this world," he said once. "Everything here is too temporary."

Terry eventually found employment as a security guard, which was enough like police work to satisfy some of his needs, and many years after that he set up his own security business, using retired police officers (of all people). Terry's transition from work to retirement was long and painful. It could have been much easier and quicker if he had been able to accept reality better, or if he could have identified his grief feelings better, or if he didn't hold in his feelings as much as he did, or even if he had sought professional help sooner. Any and all of these differences could have shortened his process.

Admittedly, few of us lose work in as early and as traumatic a way as Terry. Yet, Terry is a good example in the extreme of how a person can idolize work, a tendency that is compounded by the dynamics of bereavement. Idolizing work is easy to do in our work-oriented society, which tends to define and measure people by their work.[14] Finding sources of worth and identity apart from work is difficult. Although Terry's case is extreme in one sense, in another sense there is a Terry in all of us. We all can fall prey to the temptation to make our work into an idol. It is an issue we all must deal with in making the transition to retirement, in adjusting to the loss of work.

DOING AND BEING

When work, retirement, and aging are discussed, inevitably the distinction between doing and being surfaces. Writers who make this distinction point out that Western culture is oriented toward doing rather than being. Western culture values productivity over relation-ships. Two illustrations of this preference are issues of self-definition and self-worth. We define ourselves more by what we do, than by who we are. In response to the question, "Who are you?" we often answer, "I am a plumber," "I am a dentist," or "I am a scientist." Such statements do not say who we are so much as they say what we do. In traditional gender roles, this preference of doing over being is more typical of Western males. Daniel J. Levinson, in his 1986 study of the developmental stages of adult males, noted the importance that men attach to their work not just as a self-definition, but also as an organizing principle around which they mark their developmental stages.[15]

Similarly, the culture's definitions of worth are also linked to cate-gories of doing. We equate productivity with value. When we work, we are valuable. Those who do not work are deemed as having less value. This assumption—that busy is better—is not linked so much to gender per se. Women who are homemakers may measure themselves by how useful they are around the house or how busy they are. Older women complain loudly that they are no longer useful, because they cannot help out. The issue is more linked to the culture's traditional affection for the Protestant work ethic.

Further, writers like to point out that more traditional cultures or this culture in former centuries was more "being" oriented. In response to the inquiry, "Who are you?" people might answer from that mode, "I am your uncle," "I am a father," or "I am an African American." These are self-definitions that define us by who we are, by our relationships to other humans. Similarly, worth is linked with our place in the family or in the culture, not with what we produce.

In a culture that is heavily oriented toward the doing mode, it is hard for older adults to retire. Retirees feel useless, of less value, because they no longer produce or earn a paycheck. Speaking to this point, Eugene Bianchi writes:

> The challenge of old people from today's world is, in summary, to preserve and enhance human dignity in a hostile environment . . . they are particularly burdened and rejected in a society that focuses almost exclusively on doing over being. . . . In a society where the production of things is paramount, people are easily treated as things, to be discarded when no longer useful.[16]

Catholic theologian and mystic, Henri J. M. Nouwen, has also been particularly articulate on this point, although Nouwen labels the distinction as one between "being" and "having." Calling old age the "last segregation," Nouwen argues that this segregation occurs partly because retirees are alienated from a culture that is dominated by the values of production. It is trying for older retired adults to feel worthwhile in a culture that overemphasizes doing modes of value and worth. "The fear of becoming old in our Western world," writes Nouwen, "is determined by the fear of not being able to live up to the expectations of an environment in which you are what you can produce, achieve, have, and keep."[17] This cultural environment makes the process of retiring and maintaining dignity and self-esteem very difficult. Or to put it in the reverse, one of the developmental tasks of this stage of life, if one is to age well through this period, must be to develop and enhance self-worth, to find and affirm a self-worth that is rooted in being modes of value.

THEOLOGY OF WORK AND PLAY

This brief chapter in this small book is no place to begin a discussion of the theology of work. However, it seems to me that the nature of work is badly misunderstood in this society, and that as such it causes people a great deal of hardship at the time or retirement. It would be timely for the church to offer a vision of "good work," of how work was meant to be. Let me offer some suggestive comments along these lines.[18]

In traditional Christian thinking, work is understood as either a punishment for sin or a way to avoid sinning. The Genesis story tells us that when humankind sinned and fell out of grace, one of the consequences was having to work by "sweat of your face" (Gen 3:19). In this image of work, work is negative, laborious, and necessary. In contrast, early Protestant theology understood work as good, but its goodness was in its activity. Work is good because humans are supposed to be busy. Idleness is the breeding ground for sin. Therefore it is important to keep busy. It did not matter so much at what—just keep busy. These two ideas—work as a curse and work as an antidote for sin—have molded our cultural attitude toward work.[19] In both cases work is something people have to do, not something they want to do. Certainly, for most people in most places, this is how work is experienced. Yet, work can be and was meant to be something more.

A theology of "good work" begins with a theology of creation. God is the Creator of the earth. God also created us in the divine image. One of the aspects of having God's image within us is that we too have the capacity to create. We, unlike other animals, can be creative. Creation has traditionally been defined as "out of nothing," in contrast to "making" which is a creating out of existing materials.

Like God, humans can genuinely "create," not just "make." Our ability to create is reflected in our love for beauty, our art, our music, and our desire to order and fashion the earth. In spite of the fall of humanity from innocence and our bondage to sin, our capacity to create remains.

So then what is work? Work is meant to be a way of creating. It is one way we humans have of co-creating with God. Work is self-expression. Work, at its best, is a form of love. Through work we express our God-given urge to create. All types of work can be self-expressive—design work, service work, manual work, intellectual work, industrial work. The type of work is not a limitation to its self-expressive character. When our work is "good work," it has this self-expressive character to it. It says who we are. Occasionally, we have all experienced work like this. There have been moments in our work histories when we have created something new, done something special, achieved something wonderful, and we have known the deep satisfaction that comes with this kind of work. Unfortunately in most industrial work settings, work is seldom experienced this way. For most people most of the time, work is experienced as having little intrinsic value. We therefore attach money to work to make it extrinsically valuable. In addition, we have attached status, friendship, and prestige to work for the same reason.

If we understand work as self-expression, then we can justifiably argue that humans need to work, not to avoid idleness and not because we are extrinsically motivated, but as a way of being truly what we are, as a way of co-creating with God. If we see work as self-expression, then it really does not matter whether we get paid or not. A paycheck is irrelevant to the true essence of work. The defining criterion of work is self-expression, not earning power. "Good work" can be any activity that is self-expressive. "Good work" is larger than just paid work. "Good work" includes all of the activities that we do throughout our lives that are self-expressive. It includes housework. It includes child care or elder care. It includes volunteer work. "Good work," God's created intention for human work, is valuable not for what it produces nor for what it earns us, but for the process of self-expression it affords us. If we understood work this way, there would be no degradation of persons in retirement. In fact, there probably would be no retirement.

The Christian doctrine of vocation hints at this same view of "good work." It suggests that God gives each of us gifts and then calls us to fulfill those gifts in certain jobs. Each of us experiences a calling, not just the ordained ministers. God calls each of us to fulfill our unique selves in a particular line of work that will allow us to express ourselves, to co-create. The distinction between an occupation and a career captures some of this sense of vocation or calling. An occupation is a job in which one "occupies" time and space. A career is an expression of our unique talents and reflects a sense of being called to or destined for such work. A career usually has more of this sense of work as self-expression. Each of us finds our own calling, our good work, only in relationship to the Creator.

If we understand work as a form of self-expression, then work and play are different versions of the same creative impulse. Work and play are not opposites, not enemies. Play is also a form of self-expression. Watch children at play for awhile. What do they do? They create. They express themselves in fantasy, in art, in drama, in building. They also work in the sense that play is rehearsal for life. Someone once said that he would love to find a job that he could play at or play that he could get paid for. Rare is the person who can work with the same joy, freedom, and self-fulfillment found in play. But isn't that what we strive for in the notion of good work? Isn't that what God wants for us? Work and play, properly understood, are different dimensions of the same divine image within us.

In our life cycle, work and play are chronologically separated. We play as children; we work as adults. Then when we retire, we are allowed to play again (but only if we worked hard to save enough money). The life cycle sequence is Play-Work-Play. Richard Bolles has suggested that we need to break out of these "three boxes of life."[20] We need to find ways to blend work and play together throughout our lives, and not segregate them. By segregating them, we make the transitions of life more difficult. By limiting play to child-hood and retirement, we allow people to be too intense about work, too tied up in the many meanings of their work, thereby setting the stage for a difficult experience when they lose work. The loss of work would not be so difficult if we learned to play during our adult years. Similarly the loss of work would not be so difficult if we had a broader vision of work that understood "retirement" as a prime time for the realization of self-expressive work.[21]

NEW CHALLENGE:
A RITUAL FOR RETIREMENT

The church seems to be ambivalent about work. On one hand it values work. After all, it keeps people from sinning and makes them responsible citizens. Yet, on the other hand, the church is appropri-ately suspicious of the culture's idolization of work, which has made materialists of us all. Perhaps this is why the church has not addressed the problem of developing an appropriate ritual for the life cycle transition called retirement. In my opinion there is a critical need for such a ritual.

A retirement ritual, especially a religious ritual, is a very attractive idea, one that could be an effective tool for helping people deal with both their grief feelings and the meanings associated with work and the loss of work. It would be a wonderful opportunity for the church to assert what it has always believed—that a person's worth can not be earned through his or her work, but must be accepted as a free gift of God's grace. Evelyn and James Whitehead, in writing about retirement as a religious ritual say:

> Worth is, finally, not in productivity. Personal value is founded in something more basic than power or responsibility or salary. It rests on the rock of God's love. The cultural phenomenon of retirement can thus serve a religious function. Separating us from accumulated credentials and accustomed "proofs of merit," it invites us to acknowledge a value in life beyond and prior to human achievement.[23]

The occasion of retirement is a timely opportunity to acknowledge again that our worth, as children of God, does not depend on whether we are productive or not. Such a rite might, as the Whiteheads suggest, announce "the good news of our uselessness." What a crucial opportunity for the church to be prophetic in a society that has increasingly defined us and measured our worth by our work. On a personal level as well, such a rite could be very liberating to all who are involved in it, freeing the retiring person from old enslaving meanings, freeing him or her to enter a new stage of spiritual growth.

Several people who have also advocated a religious retirement ritual have suggested that it also have a forward-looking dimension, not just a backward-looking dimension. As Thomas B. Robb said, we need "to focus on retirement *to* instead of *from*."[23] A religious retirement ritual should include this commissioning element. Such a ritual should commission people, not retire them. It should empower them, not encourage their passivity. It should endeavor to lure them forward into a new stage of life characterized by ministry, by service to others, and most important, by a new vision of work. Toward this end, a retirement ritual should attempt to paint a new image of work as self-expression, as service to the Lord, as joyful play. It would dematerialize work and dequantify it.

The loss of work, whether it comes at retirement or at some other point in our lives, can be a growth opportunity, a chance to spiritually move beyond our limited vision of work and to see ourselves and our worth in the larger perspective of God's love. All of this is possible, however, only if we can let go of our old work, our old view of work, and our old self-definitions and measurements of our value. We must grieve it all if we wish to move on into a still greater stage of spiritual maturity in this journey called life.

Chapter 7

The Loss of Spouse

The Lord is near to the brokenhearted, and saves the crushed in spirit.

Ps 34:18

Marriage is the most intimate of life's many relationships. The bond between husband and wife can be deep, tender, and long lasting. Thus the loss of our spouse can be one of life's most devastating emotional experiences. Nearly one half of us will have this experience; it is the price of love. Most of us do not anticipate this loss very well, even though it is so inevitable. We had hoped to "grow old together." Yet, relatively few marriages last into the seventh and eighth decades of life. Most of us must cope with the last years of life alone. The loss of a spouse is one of the most significant losses of the later years, and how we cope with this loss colors our physical, mental, and spiritual health for the remainder of our lives.

THE MULTIFACETED LOSS

Unlike any other loss, the loss of a spouse is multifaceted—a loss that can be devastating precisely because it is so comprehensive in scope. When we have been married for as long as forty or fifty years, we have spent more time being married than not. Our bond to our life partner is strong and complex. We have grown together, suffered together, worked together, and loved together. Hopefully, we have become best friends. Losing a spouse after so many years and after this kind of relationship is the most painful kind of loss. The adjustment required by this kind of loss is massive. It affects every area of one's life.

Marian was married early in life. She and Michael were high school sweethearts from a small rural town upstate. She barely finished high school herself when her first child arrived. Michael started working as a plumber's helper, and over the years, he advanced to become a journeyman plumber. They never had much in the way of material things, but they worked hard and raised four children together. By contemporary standards, Marian was a timid person, but also a loyal and dependable mother and wife. She never worked outside of the home. When Michael died at the relatively young age of forty-seven, the children were mostly adults. The transition from mother, homemaker, and wife to widow, wage earner, and single person was tough for Marian.

Within the span of what seemed like a few years, Marian was forced to make several significant changes, in fact more changes than she had made at any other period in her life. She began managing her own (now limited) money for the first time. She learned to live alone. She began working outside of the home. She had to assert herself more and not rely on others to protect her. She had to learn to socialize outside of her immediate family. All of these social, psychological, and vocational changes were forced upon Marian by the advent of one loss.

Some years later, after Marian had made many of these changes, she reflected, "I really wasn't prepared for the single life. In fact, I got married early as a young girl partly to avoid being single. It was secure going from my father's house to Michael's house. But when Michael died, I was forced to grow up in ways that I never did earlier. And . . ." with a touch of sadness, "and I now have the whole rest of my life to learn it."

One of the questions that Marian's story raises is what it is exactly that is lost in the death of a spouse. The loss of a spouse is actually composed of several losses. Certainly, we have lost the person, the unique individual that we have known and loved for many years. Moreover, we have also lost all of the roles or functions that this person fulfilled in our lives. Our spouse was a lover and sexual partner. He or she was a provider. He or she was our companion. He or she was a household manager, accountant, and a repair person. Our spouse was also a co-parent to our children. When we lose our spouse we may lose any or all of these roles as well. Each one of these losses will require adjustment and change for the survivor.

In addition, the loss of our spouse will bring with it "secondary losses." Some typical secondary losses include: loss of income, loss of home, loss of work or of a lifestyle without working. Hopefully a widowed person has some financial cushion that can mitigate some of the harshness of these secondary losses. Not every widow, however, has this kind of cushion, and some must move within months or take a job within weeks of their spouse's death. In such cases, the secondary loss may actually become more difficult to adjust to than the primary loss of a mate. When we speak of secondary losses, we also must be concerned about the cumulative effect of such losses. When losses pile upon losses, then we can become overwhelmed and potentially crippled. This is the danger that resides in the loss of spouse. The death of our spouse is unique among all of the losses in the later years, precisely because of its multifaceted character. Its scope is comprehensive.

FEMINIZATION OF DEATH

The loss of a spouse is largely a woman's issue in our culture. The vast majority of older Americans are women. Among people over sixty-five years old, 51 percent of women compared to 13 percent of men are widowed.[1] Anyone who has ever observed a random group of elderly people will notice this obvious and painful truth. Most of the time the man dies first, leaving the widowed wife to carry on without him. Men tend to die at an earlier age for a variety of psychological and physiological reasons.

Some women, particularly women who have been raised in more traditional ways, are ill-prepared to live independent lives. Yet it is the woman who is more often than not left alone after the death of a spouse. It is the woman who must learn to live independently. Few men need to make this adjustment because either they die young or they remarry more frequently and more quickly than women do. In addition, in this age of longevity, we observe that the mean duration of widowed life is approximately fourteen years for women and seven years for men.[2] Robert Hansson, Jacqueline Remondet, and Marlene Galusha have suggested, therefore, that widowhood be treated as a "career." They write:

That is, for most persons, widowhood need not be considered the end to a productive life but, rather, the beginning of a major segment of the life course, to be pursued vigorously if it is to be successful and fulfilling.[3]

As with any career, they suggest that people, particularly women, be prepared, educated, and trained for widowhood. "Personal control," they argue, is the key to success in aging well over the life span of widowhood, just as it is for one's career.

I would think that given the inevitability of spousal death and the feminization of this loss, we as a culture could do more to prepare women for this loss and its transition. Most women, in my experience, are inadequately prepared. On second thought, most men, are inadequately prepared too.

In addition, the research has demonstrated a causal link between mortality rates and bereavement. Colin Murray Parkes was one of the earliest social scientists to document this connection through his study of London widows, which concluded that during the first year of conjugal bereavement, widows are at a high risk for all kinds of illnesses, both mental and physical, including catastrophic illnesses such as cancer and heart disease.[4] In more recent times, Margaret and Wolfgang Stroebe have concluded, through their review of literature through 1990, that

> mortality risk clearly increases for the bereaved. This effect has been shown across a wide range of cultures, historical periods, types of relationships and even socioeconomic groups. We believe that the first few weeks and months are the most critical, but that substantial risk persists for longer than this period. . . . widowers are at more excessive risk than widows.[5]

The connecting causal link appears to be stress. Bereavement is, after all, stressful and therefore potentially a serious impact on the bereaved person's health and well-being.

With all of these concerns, mental, social, and physical, women need to be more thoroughly prepared for the transition from marriage to widowhood than they are. Preparation could begin with just an honest realization that for most women this loss is inevitable. It has been my experience, however, that of all of life's losses this is the one that people are least prepared for mentally, socially, and financially. Even though we know it will happen, the prevailing myths about love, romance, and marriage lead most people to avoid any serious mental or emotional preparation for this loss. So it is then that more people than not seem to be ill-prepared for the loss of their spouse.

THE UNEXPECTED LOSS

The loss of a spouse can come in many ways and forms. Probably the most difficult is through a sudden death. This is often the circumstance surrounding the death of the first spouse and it is therefore more likely to be the woman's experience of the death of her husband. The unexpected death catches us by surprise. It shatters our denial systems and illusions that "love will last forever." The unexpected loss causes us some unique emotional difficulties.[6]

Shock and disbelief are the two dominant themes in the early responses to sudden loss. The psychological shock we experience is not unlike the physical shock that our bodies go through when faced with a similar sudden physical trauma. The function is the same. The purpose of shock is to shut down the psyche, "to pull the circuit breaker," and to turn off the power. We are overloaded. We cannot cope with that much pain and trauma all at once. So our psyches shut down. Time out!

Most people experience a numbing effect right after they hear the news of an unexpected death. In Lifton's classic study of the survivors of the atomic blast at Hiroshima, he described shock as "psychic numbing" and said that people just "ceased to feel."[7] Emotionally, sudden deaths feel as traumatic as a nuclear bomb blast. We can be just as shocked. When we are in shock, we tune out emotionally. We walk about in a daze, preoccupied, or in what one person called "a mild trance." People talk and we mumble something back. We say, "I can't believe this is happening." "No, not me! Not now! Not my Jim." "Not my Alice!" That is disbelief and shock.

Mel's wife died suddenly in a car accident. She was in her early sixties, as was her husband. Mel experienced all of the classic shock symptoms. He noted some months later, "You know, Pastor, the thing that really helped me the most to come to terms with Marge's death was the viewing. Not too many people came to the viewing. I guess people don't like those things these days—but it sure helped me. There is nothing like the cold, dead body of your wife to help you really realize that she is dead. I must have sat there for hours, most of the time alone. It took that long—but gradually it sunk in: 'She's dead, Mel. She is dead!'" Rituals can be tools, as in Mel's case, to help widowed spouses break through the shock and disbelief. They also can help reinforce denial. Much depends on how the ritual is structured and conducted.

Shock can last for a few hours or several days. Gradually, it gives way to panic, emotional release, and anger. Disbelief now alternates more frequently with periods of weeping, mourning, and emotional release. Soon we have entered the full throes of our grief work. When death comes unexpectedly, grief is usually very intense, very volatile. There was little time to prepare ourselves emotionally. There was no time for anticipatory grief. Like it or not, we are thrust into a process we cannot control or avoid. The only way out is through.

Often when a spouse dies unexpectedly, the last time we were together becomes very important. We remember vividly the last scene, the last words, the last embrace. Every detail is vivid in our memory. The colors, sounds, place, the touch of his or her hand, the subtle meanings that only we know. It is as though somebody pressed the "freeze" button on the VCR and the movie of our life froze at this last scene.

If our last memory of our beloved spouse was pleasant, then we are indeed fortunate. We have a nice memory to comfort us in our sorrow. Many other people are not so fortunate. Perhaps they were not able to be present when the spouse died and they wanted to be. Perhaps in that last conversation they wanted to say something more, but didn't. Or perhaps the last conversation was an argument or a negative exchange. They left feeling unfinished, saying to themselves, "I'll straighten this out tomorrow," but unfortunately, tomorrow never comes. Or perhaps they made a promise that they couldn't fulfill. All of these things can now be haunting our souls.

If the frozen "last scene" of our beloved spouse is negative, then in our sorrow we must work to soften these mental images. If we are to grieve well, we must do some intentional editing of our mental movie. Erase those negative scenes, if they are such. Choose to go back to an earlier time, prior to the last contact, and focus on another scene that you feel is more representative of how you feel about your deceased spouse or one that is more representative of your relationship as a whole. Focus on that scene. Dwell on it. Allow it to comfort you and speak to you in your sorrow.

What strikes people so forcibly in the case of the sudden or unexpected loss is the finality of it all. He or she is gone now. Our beloved sweetheart whom we have known most of our lives is gone, is suddenly nowhere to be found. There isn't anywhere on the entire face of the earth where we can go to find him or her. We can't call our spouse on the phone. We can't pretend that he or she is just out of town for a while. He or she is gone now, and somehow, some way, we must find the strength to go on.

LOSS BY DIVORCE

The loss of one's spouse can come not only by death, but also by divorce. Divorce is nothing new. In the past fifty years or so, we have seen a significant increase in the number of divorces in our society. Many of these divorces come early in the life of the marriage and are followed by a second marriage. Yet, for the woman who divorces late in life, say over the age of fifty, the probability of remarriage is relatively small. This is less true for men, given the realities of the sex ratios of the population and the preferred age differentials between men and women[8], "The dream" dies hard, to quote a term from *Flying Solo: Single Women in Midlife*.[9] For all intents and purposes divorce is "as good as a death." She will probably live the rest of her life alone. That is harsh news for most women. The fantasy of remarriage dies hard.

Beverly was fifty-four years old when her marriage dissolved. It had been dead for many years prior to that. There was little communication, no sexual intimacy, and no cooperation on even basic household decisions. Max had long ago set up a separate bank account for himself, leaving Beverly with the joint account. Beverly had taken a part-time job as a payroll clerk some years earlier, which later evolved into a full-time position after the divorce. "I suppose that we just stayed together out of convenience," said Bev. "It was easier than anything else." In those last few years of the marriage, however, Max began to be abusive, not just verbally as he had always been, but physically abusive. In addition, he formed a relationship with a younger woman and went out of his way to flaunt it in Beverly's face. All of this finally pushed Beverly to file for divorce. Convenience was no longer worth it.

Whether she knew it or not at the time, Beverly had entered the next stage of her life. Initially she had fantasies about remarriage someday, but objectively the prospects were not good. She had gained considerable weight in later years and was by her own admission very "plain" looking. She was a down-to-earth "den mother type." She was hardly the type for the single's bars, and as a life-long Catholic, she soon came to realize that "one marriage was enough for her."

Beverly's experience of the loss of her spouse was considerably different from the person who loses a beloved spouse through death. For Beverly there was little grief and sorrow. Her mourning was colored more by anger, despair, and feelings of helplessness. She had years of resentful feelings toward Max, most of which were internalized into self-blame and depression. Yet for Beverly the hardest part was just learning to live alone, learning to do so many things for herself. She didn't miss Max per se, but she did miss the married life, the home, and having "a man around the house." Sometimes she would joke and say, "I'm going to get me a six-foot cardboard poster of Paul Newman to place in the corner of the kitchen, so that I can have a man around the house. That was about as much good as Max ever was anyhow."

What Beverly's story reminds us of is that the loss of a spouse can come in ways other than death. Beverly also reminds us that not all grief work is sad. Sometimes grief includes powerful feelings of anger, resentment, and despair. These feelings must also be worked through if one is to be able to let go of the past and move on to the next phase of life.

LONELINESS

The initial throes of grief are demanding, painful, and horrible. Some people say that the first month is the worst. Pain and agony dominate our lives, consume our energy, and take up most of our waking time and sometimes our sleeping hours. These are the times when family support is most crucial and useful. It is helpful to have relatives and family present. They can carry us through the initial days and weeks, making decisions, completing chores, notifying relatives, and taking care of some of the unpleasant chores that accompany a funeral and burial.

What most widowed people experience, however, is that family support gives way within a few days or weeks. Sooner or later, and usually it's sooner, the widowed person is left alone. Now we are really alone perhaps for the first time since our spouse's death. Now we feel the depth of our loneliness. Returning to that empty house, sleeping in the empty bed, setting a place for one at the dinner table—these are some of the little things, and there are many more as well, that rub salt in the wound of grief. These are the things that remind us that we are truly alone. Our pain reaches a new depth, an existential depth that rattles the very foundations of our soul.

Loneliness is the most difficult of the long-term problems of widowhood. The grief wound will heal in time, but loneliness is a mental state that will not heal. After grief is done, Dr. Feinberg says:

> There remains loneliness. This is a longer range result, which is not susceptible to the same healing process. Loneliness is the reaction to the absence of the valued relationship rather than to the experience of the loss. Every other aspect of grief may subside as time goes on, but as long as no new relationship is formed to replace the one that is lost, loneliness continues.[10]

Loneliness, however, can be cared for, and caring does much to help widowed people cope with the loneliness.[11] Loneliness is not usually cured, except in forming a new love relationship. Some people will do that, but for most others in later life, that cannot or will not happen. They must learn to live with loneliness.

LEARNING TO REACH OUT

Social isolation is slightly different from, but related to, the problem of loneliness. Social isolation is usually defined as being isolated from a social network of friends, family, work colleagues, etc. Most widowed people discover that they are both lonely and socially isolated after their spouse dies. Most widowed people discover that once they are widowed, their social network changes dramatically. Many of their couple friends gradually cease calling or visiting. Associates of the deceased spouse, work colleagues and friends also fade away in time. Perhaps they are uncomfortable because you remind them of their loss. Perhaps you remind them of their own mortality. For whatever reason, widowed people become more socially isolated with time.

Most widowed people try to socialize. They are told that they need to get out of the house. It is difficult at first, because they are so used to doing things as part of a pair. It is hard going to restaurants and movies alone or to church and sit alone. These are awkward activities to do at first, and every time we do it, we are reminded again that we are alone. Yet, the advice givers are correct. Our mental health does depend on how much we socialize, on how well we can rebuild a network of support for ourselves.[12]

As the years pass, our circle of friends shifts more and more to people our own age and status. This is not entirely desirable, but other widowed people do understand our feelings more than most others. In time we may even relocate, giving up the larger family home for smaller quarters designed for a single person. If we relocate due to health reasons, we may reexperience the pain of being alone. We never wanted to be alone. It was never our wish to spend our later years without our life partner. We may wish that our spouse was here all the more. Being lonely is bad enough, "but to be old and lonely is the pits," as one friend of mine said recently. I would add, "Being old, lonely, and poor is the absolute worst." This is the plight of many our elderly citizens. Loneliness and social isolation are facts of life for the older single person. The loss of spouse is the event that ushers in this predicament, and from that point on we must learn to live with loneliness.

In spite of the fact that social isolation increases with age and dramatically increases after the death of our spouse, we can and must work hard at learning to reach out. Social support, family, and friendships, even involvement in larger issues of the world, are important ingredients in staying youthful in the later years.[13] In fact I argue, as does Eugene C. Bianchi, that this is the spiritual developmental task of late life, learning to stay involved. He writes:

Elderhood, therefore, is not a time to withdraw from the world, but rather to make a special offering to fellow humans through a deeper involvement in the worldly sphere. We do not agree that "the last time is for oneself" . . . we have stressed the theme of an old age more fully committed to the great needs of humanity.[14]

Obviously not everyone stays active, nor can everyone, because of physical limitations. (Being involved is as much a state of mind as it is a physical state.) Some people are just overwhelmed by the progressive losses of later life and prefer to gradually withdraw from life. Nevertheless, I believe that this is an important developmental task of later life and a task that is ushered upon us when our spouse dies. Learning to reach out, learning to stay involved in life, requires that we first learn to grieve well.

In Chapter 6, we discussed the loss of friends that occurs when a person retires from his or her life's work. Many friendships are built around work and work activities. When we retire, those routine social contacts no longer occur automatically. In retirement, we have to be more intentional about making and maintaining our friendships. The point is worth repeating again in the context of spousal bereavement. Friendships were often easier to maintain when married, because most of our socializing was done as a couple. Now that we are alone, we must be intentional about friendships. We must go out of our way to make and keep friends. Learning to reach out is one of the key ingredients in our successful adjustment to this post-marriage period of life. Yet, "reaching out" is not possible psychologically until we have grieved the passing of our spouse.

LEARNING SELF-SUFFICIENCY

One of the central themes that I hear from widowed people is that they must learn to be independent and self-reliant again. Moreover, if they have never really been on their own, then they must learn self-reliance for the first time. There are hundreds of little things that we have relied on our spouse to do for us. Now we must do them all.

Most people who have been married a long time grow to be dependent on their spouse. This is part of the nature of marriage. Even the most independent person usually grows more dependent as the years go by. We have become accustomed to being dependent, psychologically, financially, and even physically. Then when our spouse dies, we are suddenly without our usual source of support. For some people that process will be relatively easy, for others, it will be much more difficult.

Olive cried with tears of frustration as well as loss. This was the fourth time that she had the Buick in the shop for those squeaky brakes. It was so frustrating. She felt that she was being given "the run around." Yet she knew so little about cars. That was Truman's hobby. He used to keep the cars humming. "Now that he's gone," Olive complained, "I have to do all this myself and I don't know a darn thing about cars. God help me if I ever break down on the highway."

Learning to do things on our own can be one of the more difficult adjustments of widowhood. Whatever our spouse used to do for us, we must now do for ourselves (or at least arrange to get outside help). Did she wash clothes? Now you must learn to do it. Did he do the taxes every year? Now you must. Did she keep the gardens weeded? Now you must. Did he paint the house every summer? Now you must assume that assignment. Eventually, we will have to reduce our responsibilities, not expand them. But as long as we are able, we must assume new roles. We must become more self-reliant. We can do it if we take it easy and look upon it as a challenge. We may not be able to do these things as well as our spouse did, and that's okay too. We are learning.

For Jess, money was one of those areas that Darlene had always taken charge of. He just gave her his paycheck every two weeks. He probably had not written a check in ten years. But now he had to learn the ropes. In fact, now that she was gone, he had a strong urge to put his life in order. He wanted to see the old tax returns and review the insurance policies and update his will. He wanted to get things settled, so the kids knew exactly what to do when he passed on. In addition he knew that he would be living on a reduced income in the next few years. He had to start managing his money now, otherwise it wouldn't last. He didn't want to end up like his mother, poor and sick, in some state warehouse for the elderly.

"I've had a funny desire to put my house in order since Darlene died," he told me. "I guess I am preparing for my own death or something like that. I want to take inventory of my life, see what I got, and how long it can last me. If I live as long as my mother, I'll go broke—unless I learn to manage money."

"Will you?" I asked.

"Certainly. Old dogs can learn new tricks," Jess affirmed. "Just watch me."

AVOID MAKING IDOLS

Most widowed people, particularly in the early stages of grief, cling to the memory of their beloved partner. They resist letting go. They may even idealize the lost spouse. If we do not grieve in a proper and timely fashion, then this tendency to idealize the deceased becomes exaggerated. It turns into idolization, which works to block our natural grieving process and keep us stuck in the past.

Jean, forty-six, was married to John, a noted physician in the community. After John's untimely death, Jean seemed to grieve well enough, but in time the grief did not subside. By two years after her husband's death, Jean had made a little shrine to her deceased husband in his former office/study. Photographs, trophies, and awards were everywhere—from certificates of merit from the American Medical Association to the first place trophy at the local YMCA bowling tournament. He had been a very popular and active man who made many friends and contacts in the medical community. When visitors came to call on Jean, she would show them all through his study, like a tour guide in the museum, only she added tears at all the right spots. In time, visitors came less often, but the shrine lived on.

I had the opportunity to talk with Jean's adult children, who expressed great concern for their mother's lack of resolution of their father's death. The children visited her less often now themselves. They were increasingly uncomfortable with their mother's "tour." In fact, they were beginning to resent what their mother was doing to their father. "We don't recognize the man mother has created," they told me one day. "Mom has turned Dad into a saint or something. We hardly recognize him. To us he was an ordinary guy. He swore and he had a bad temper, but he was our dad. This fellow that she has plastered about the walls—that's not Dad; that is some Greek god!"

"Mom hasn't let Dad go," one of the daughters continued. "She is still trying to keep him alive. I wish she would let him die. For God's sake, let him rest in peace."

Widowed people can, just like people grieving any loss, make what was lost into a false god. It starts with idealizing the beloved spouse. They gloss over his or her mistakes and faults. They remember the lovely, tender, wonderful moments. All of this is normal enough. Everyone idealizes the departed, especially if one enjoyed a good relationship with the spouse. Yet if people get stuck there, then they have made their spouse into a mini-god. They have started to worship at the shrine instead of at the altar of the living God.

One way to get at the issue of idolatry is by examining the beliefs that inform one's operational theology. By so examining, we can often see clearly that an individual has constructed a theology that is based on a false god. Jean was very consumed with her husband's success long before he died. She lived by the belief that "I am worthwhile because I am married to a successful man." Her identity was his identity. Her worth was in his success. She came to glorify in his success, as if it was her own. When John died, she never challenged that belief; she just rearranged it to read: "I am worthwhile because I was married to a successful man." So she continued to glory in his success. In fact, in her grieving the story got more exaggerated.

Jean's story reminds us of another common belief, a more generalized belief, that many widowed people affirm. This creed reads: "The happiest time of my life was when I was married." Sounds innocent enough, doesn't it? Most of us, especially if we had good marriages, agree with this statement. Yet, it can be a destructive belief if carried to the extreme. Such an assumption can prevent us from seeing the possibilities for happiness in the present moment. Surely in the midst of our grief we have all said, "Life is meaningless now," or "There is nothing for me now," or "I cannot go on without him or her," and so on. But we did not get stuck there. We did not start to believe that salvation is found only in the past—or did we?

Fortunately, Jean got some help for her idolatry, and through therapy, individually and with her children, she was able to let go of her fierce loyalty to her husband. Her new life began to emerge when she was elected to the board of directors of the local community hospital. At first it was an honorary position, partly out of respect for her deceased husband, but in time she made the "calling" her own. She poured herself into fund-raising, community outreach programs, and employee relations. She was a model board member, giving time and energy beyond all bounds.

She went on to live thirty years after her husband died. They were good years, filled with purpose, service to others, and self-worth. When she finally "retired" there was a testimonial dinner at the hospital, not for John's wife, but for Jean: community leader, humanitarian, and volunteer par excellence. She had reordered her life and her theology. Her operational creed now read, "I am worthwhile because I do worthwhile things." Not a perfect belief, but much more healthy than her former creed.

Each stage of life is valuable in its own right and the post-marriage stage of life can be valuable too. In many ways it may be the most valuable. God has a plan for each of us during this time, just as God had purposes for each stage of our lives up to this point. We are still alive for a reason and we are alone for a reason. We need to find these reasons and "work out our salvation with fear and trembling" (Phil 2:12). The years we spent with our husband or wife were good years, hopefully. The present years can also be good—maybe a different kind of good, but still good. For this goodness to emerge, we must first grieve.

CHANGING IDENTITIES

Few other losses in later life alter our identity as much as the loss of our spouse. It used to be "we," but now it is "I." We feel stripped. We feel lonely. We feel incomplete. We pass through an identity crisis not unlike our earlier one in adolescence.

Yet in a broader sense, changes to our identity are inevitable with every loss of the later years. After all, our identity is built around who and what we are emotionally attached to. We define ourselves by our roles. "I am a mother" . . . "a florist". . . . "an Englishman". . . . "a widow." We are our roles. . . . and yet as we have repeatedly noted, in the second half of life each one of our major roles, and many of the minor ones, are lost to us. With each loss, then, we must redefine ourselves. Each loss brings with it a small identity crisis, "Who am I now? . . . now that I am alone?. . . "now that I am no longer a parent?" . . . "now that I am no longer a worker?" . . . now that I am no longer whole?"

With each loss of later life, comes a corresponding loss of identity or change of identity. As we age, we are regularly losing pieces of our identity, which may or may not be replaced with new pieces. For some this will be a problem, because they have formed an identity largely around one role or one attachment. Those who have a variety of roles will weather the storm easier.

When we look at the aging process as a whole, we can liken the repeated loss of identities as a kind of "kenosis" experience. Like an onion, some feel that each loss strips away another layer of the self, forcing us to dig deeper into the self, leading in time to the individual's core identity, the one single identity under all of the layers. In this sense, aging with its repeated losses can be an opportunity for deep spiritual growth, because the successive losses of roles and attachments forces us to search for a deeper definition of self, an identity that transcends all other identities.

There is considerable debate in the field of gerontology concerning the role religion plays in the life of the elderly. Do older people become more religious as they age? Research that measures religious sentiment according to objective criteria, such as attendance at religious services, argues that older people are not more religious. Others argue that the approaching personal crisis of death forces older people to think more about the ultimate meanings of life, thus they become more religious.

My view is that older people, generally speaking, can and do become more spiritual in the second half of life. My view is that the second half of life is essentially a spiritual journey, precisely because it involves the kenosis process that I described. The second half of life is filled with powerful and repeated loss experiences. Each one of those losses forces us to let go of some beloved attachment or role. In that letting go, we must now dig deeper for an definition of ourselves that transcends these various losses.

Increasingly, we are drawn to self-definitions that are based on spiritual criteria or "internal" criteria, instead of external criteria. We start defining ourselves by who we are, not what we do, or how we look, or what we own or who we were married to. Most of the losses described in this book are losses of things external . . . our looks, our health, our children, our work, our home, and our spouse. Thus, with each of these losses, we are driven to define ourselves more and more by "internal" criteria, criteria of character, instead of criteria of production, of appearance, of possession, or even of relationship.

Each loss in the later years is painful. None is more painful than the loss of one's spouse, especially if that marriage has been a happy one and long one. The loss of one's spouse forces us to come to terms with our identity in a deeper way. It forces us to let go of the "we," and squarely and painfully face the "I." Who am I apart from my marriage? Apart from the many roles I played in that relationship? Apart from my various attachments? Many people find this transition from plural to singular very painful and certainly very lonely. Yet, there can be a hidden benefit in this process. A keener sense of the "I" might lead to a new, stronger, and more durable definition of self. And often, for the fortunate few that realize this benefit, the deeper identity that they reach for is one rooted in the spiritual or the internal criteria. Such an identity can weather the loss of spouse, and only such an identity can transcend all the losses of the later years.

LETTING GO, AGAIN

As we get older, it seems more and more difficult to let go completely of past losses, with loss of spouse one of the most difficult to relinquish. The loss of spouse demands so many significant adjustments in our lifestyle, roles, and attitudes. It is a painful loss to grieve. It is so tempting to think that happiness can be found only by going backward, not forward. And so, while we do not make little shrines to our dead spouse, neither do we live fully in the present. We long for the past. The living God, however, is not in the past, but always pulling us toward a new life in the future. So, we must again let go, knowing that the invisible arms of the Almighty will support us and carry us forward to a new stage of our journey through life.

Chapter 8

The Loss of Health

So do not lose heart. Though our outer nature is wasting away, our inner nature is being renewed every day.

I Cor 4:16

One of the inevitable losses faced in later life is the gradual loss of health. All of us will experience this loss unless we die unexpectedly at an early age. For most of us there is no single, sudden loss of health. The loss of health is experienced as a gradual decline, peppered with many points of realization when we are keenly aware of what we have lost. Actually, we might say that the loss of health is really many losses, all strung together over the years. With each loss in health or realization thereof, we must learn to modify our lifestyle to accommodate our new limitations or ailments. Some of us make modifications easily. Others get caught up in denial or feelings of bitterness or despair. Dealing with the loss of health becomes a perpetual theme in the second half of life.

THE FIRST EXPERIENCE OF THIS LOSS

As a part of my health maintenance program, I do a little jogging. In the process of participating in various running events in recent years, I have noticed that the largest number of participants are always in the age range of forty to fifty-five years. The competition for medals among these categories of runners is fierce. Not too many younger competitors. Not too many older competitors. I suppose the older people are not present in large numbers because running gets to be an increasingly stressful sport for older bodies. The younger people are not present in large numbers because they are still taking their health for granted. So, why are the middle-aged men and women there in force?

In almost every case when I have talked at length to middle-aged runners, I find that these people are unusually aware of the fragile nature of their health. Typically, they have some "horror story" that illustrates this point. The conclusion of the story is always, ". . . and that's what started me running." I have speculated therefore that middle age is about the time that many people first experience a loss in health. This loss is relatively minor, compared to the losses that will come later in life, but the novelty of this first loss has a powerful effect. It motivates some people to get involved in exercise in a very serious way.

This first loss or first awareness of loss is often a very powerful experience precisely because it is our first realization that our health is declining. The existential quality of this first loss of health shakes the foundations of our life. Furthermore, how we react to this, the first health loss, often sets the pattern for how we will respond to the many losses of health that follow. We have a choice between facing reality and evasion. How we choose this time, more than in the times to follow, determines the direction of our spiritual journey.

The actual loss or realization of loss can occur in hundreds of ways, large and small. Some people experience this first loss in very dramatic ways. Perhaps they have a heart attack or develop a chemical dependency or lose a body part in an accident. Now they are forced to make radical adjustments in their lifestyle, in their diet, in their daily routine, in their priorities and their attitudes. These adjustments will be preceded by some difficult emotional dynamics. Sudden losses do get our attention. They are hard to deny. Yet the sudden nature of the change can be overwhelming. Most of us will need time to process our feelings, change our attitudes, and then modify our behaviors. If we have been caught by surprise, then these adjustments will take some time.

For most people this first realization of the loss of health usually comes in "smaller," more subtle ways. Can you remember when you first realized your body was declining? Perhaps you realized one Monday morning, as your muscles ached with pain, that you just can't play tennis once a month and expect to perform as usual. Or perhaps you have thrown your back out for the third time this year after trying to move furniture. Or perhaps your physician has just had a serious talk with you about your forty extra pounds or your high blood pressure. Or perhaps you've discovered that you are a borderline diabetic and it runs in the family.

Typically, these kinds of changes first get noticed when we are in our forties or fifties. Yet it is hard to say exactly when and where this first realization of the loss of health comes. It is largely an individual experience. Some of us can be very good at ignoring the many "clues" that our bodies offer us. We flee from the frightening feelings and implications embedded in those clues. This is the first awareness of the loss of health.

CHANGING OUR ASSUMPTIONS ABOUT LIFE

The loss of health is tied closely with our own finitude which is also a common theme during the midlife years and beyond. It is related therefore to the loss of youth, which was discussed in Chapter 3.[1] We first experience our finitude not in any direct encounter with death, but in the bumping up against our own limitations. This realization of our limitations can be experienced in several areas of life during the later years. We might experience limits in our career, and/or in our finances, and/or in our emotional life, and, of course, in our health. The loss of health can be understood as a part of this larger experience of "bumping up against the limits" that becomes more common as we pass the midpoint of life.

Part of the uniqueness of the loss of health in the second half of life, as compared to life's first half, is that these losses of health are now permanent. Increasingly we are dealing with changes in our health that are permanent or semipermanent conditions. Up to this point in our lives, our occasional physical limitations have been temporary. We get sick and we get well. We break a leg and it heals. We are tired and we rest. We experience distresses in our bodies as temporary. We remember so well our mother's sweet assurance, "Tomorrow you'll be as good as new." Our operational belief about illness is that "this too will pass." Most of us have never had to learn to deal with permanent limitations—until now.

The finality of these losses is new and challenges our basic assumptions about life and health. Initially most of us do not realize that this change has taken place. We respond to illness or limitations as if they can be fixed and then we can go on with life as usual. Unknown to us, the rules of the game of life have changed.

Jim's experience with hypertension was like this. When his doctor first told him that his blood pressure was dangerously high, he was concerned. He had never had high blood pressure before, but he had read about the potentially dangerous effects of chronic high blood pressure in magazines and health journals. He was appropriately alarmed. Jim's first response was to try to cure it. He lost twenty pounds, began exercising daily, and watched his stress levels. Sure enough, the blood pressure went down. He fixed it—so he thought. Then over the following months, Jim again got busy at work and began to be less faithful with his new health regime. Two years later, at his regular checkup, the blood pressure was back up there again, as high as ever. Again he began exercising, and he again was able to lower the numbers. This time, however, he monitored the situation more carefully, almost scientifically. Jim noticed that as soon as he let up, even just a little, the blood pressure rose that next month. That's when it really hit Jim. A new realization began to surface in his consciousness: he wasn't ever going to cure his blood pressure problem. It was here to stay, for the rest of his life. The problem was permanent, final. This was a hard concept to accept at first. He had to change his way of thinking about health, from viewing physical problems as temporary, to beginning to see them as permanent. Only as Jim made this conceptual change (I would say, change in operational theology) did his response to the blood pressure change too. To effectively deal with the blood pressure problem, his behavioral changes needed to be as permanent as the condition. He needed a response that matched the new reality.

Another of these operational beliefs associated with the loss of health that Jim's story illustrates is the assumption that our body will take care of itself. In the past when we were young, our body did take care of itself to a great extent. It developed automatically. It seemed to recover from illness or injury well enough. There was usually a parenting figure watching out for our body, of course. Nevertheless, for the most part, our bodies seemed to heal themselves. There seemed to be an underlying thrust toward health and growth.

Now, post-midlife, the situation has changed. Our bodies do not automatically take care of themselves. In fact, we now see something quite frightening. We see that the natural inclination of the body is decline. If we just leave the body alone, as we always have done, it will not stay neutral; it will gradually decline. Think about it! Gradually, most of us gain weight with increased age. Our blood pressure rises. Our arteries harden with each passing year. Our muscles become more weak and inflexible as we age. All this is as normal as growth was in childhood. Decline is as inevitable as health was through the first half of life. "A new level of brokenness is experienced," writes Eugene Bianchi, as we realize the inevitability of this decline of health.[2]

Linda passed her fortieth birthday in good spirits because she had gotten on an exercise "kick" about a year before. She did not feel old. In fact, in some ways she was in the best shape of her life. Yet she could see that the direction of her body's processes had changed. "Up to this point," she noted, "you can be lousy to your body and get away with it, but from here on, you must take care of it. Eat right. Exercise. If not, it's all downhill."

This realization is very hard for some of us to perceive, and when we do, our souls cry out with St. Paul that the whole creation is in "bondage to decay" and we long for the "redemption of our bodies" (Rom 8:21-23). It is a frightening prospect, this decline. Yet we must face it. It is the truth. Only if we realize that the ground rules of life have changed can we then begin to deal with our health constructively. Only then can we modify our attitudes, our theological assumptions; and our lifestyles accordingly.

Another way of saying the same thing is that from here on we must be "proactive" regarding our health. In the past we could afford to be "reactive" to health problems. When it broke, we fixed it; and "if it isn't broken, don't fix it." Now we cannot afford to continue that response pattern. Actually, at this stage of our lives we can probably be as healthy as we have ever been if we work at it. We certainly do not need to be old and sickly. The difference is that now we must work at it. We must take responsibility for maintaining our health, because the rules of the game have changed.

RESPONSES TO THE LOSS OF HEALTH

Obviously many people do not make this shift in attitude from a reactive to a proactive stance toward their health. Just look around.

Many people middle age and older gain weight year after year, smoke until it kills them, and ignore their doctor's advice about diet even when their health problem is staring them in the face. These people are largely denying their loss of health.

Denial is probably the most common way of responding to the loss of health. The initial health losses are so gradual and subtle that it is relatively easy to go on pretending that we can do everything that we used to do. Other people cling to denial even after their bodies have started to dysfunction and even after their physicians have given them explicit instructions regarding how to treat their ailment. Denial can be fatal.

Many people respond to the loss of health with despair, especially after repeated attempts to fix their problem. Such people seem to resign themselves to the gradual decline of their health. They seem to adopt a fatalistic attitude. Yes, they periodically make token efforts to bolster their health on a reactive basis, but their efforts are short-lived. They "believe" that they are fighting a losing battle, that in this life death is victorious. Such people are often helpless and passive and seem to be just waiting for their time. This despairing response to the loss of health is rare in the early years of later life, but it becomes increasingly more common as we observe people in later and later stages of life.

Another common response to the loss of health is anger and bitterness. It is such a shock to many people when they realize that their health is fading, that their bodies now require time and intentionality. Some people feel betrayed by their bodies, others feel estranged. Their bodies used to be so predictable, so trustworthy. Most of us are not accustomed to having physical limitations. Anger and frustration can be a normal, emotional response to the loss of health.

Pamela was fifty-four years old when she was diagnosed as having irritable bowel syndrome. Actually, she had had digestive problems for the past ten years, but they were easy to ignore. It was simple enough to "cure" the immediate problem, but over the long term, her doctor told her that she must watch her diet. No more spicy foods. No more coffee. No more onions. No more Mexican salsa. No more alcohol. It was interesting to counsel with Pam over the following three to five years and observe her cyclical pattern of denial and anger. She would follow her doctor's orders for a while and her digestive tract would be

OK. Then she would cheat a little bit—onions on a hamburger here, a few cups of coffee there—just "to prove that she could still do it." And sure enough, within the day she was crippled over with pain and rushing to the bathroom with diarrhea. Again she would get some medicine and work hard to calm down her bowels and stomach. A few months later, however, the pattern would repeat itself. This cycle actually went on for years. As Pamela described it, she felt angry, "cheated" that she couldn't eat the way she used to. She just couldn't believe that she could never drink a glass of wine again, and so she'd try again and again to prove reality different than it was. And again her body would prove to her that things had changed. She would seem to accept her condition, then in anger try to prove that it wasn't so. Eventually, as she learned to grieve and let go, she accepted her loss of health and made the necessary changes in her lifestyle.

HEALTH AND SALVATION

I have suggested that when grief feelings are not worked through, one of the results can be a kind of idolatry wherein the person comes to worship that which is lost. Such people become fixated on the lost object—in this case, health—and believe in their deepest souls that they can have it back and keep it forever if they just work hard enough. Or to put it differently, the false god promises the worshiper a kind of salvation—in this case perpetual health.

Have you known people who seem to have idolized their health and its maintenance? I certainly have. They are found most often in health food stores, in health spas, in tanning salons, and at the vitamin counters. Nothing is wrong with such measures when they are done within reason, but the "true believer" does not practice moderation. The idol's demands are total or nothing at all. They become preoccupied, even obsessed with their bodies. They can act like hypochondriacs, talking incessantly about their symptoms. Health worshipers believe (and I use that word intentionally) that their salvation lies in the maintenance of their health. In fact, the health worshiper comes to equate health with salvation. They are one and the same in the mind of the worshiper. The unspoken illusion is that if I can maintain my health in a perfected state, then death, decline, and disease can be held at bay or at least controlled.[3]

Health worshipers can be any age. They are more obvious and numerous during middle age, because health does seem to be more controllable then. The lure of the false god is plausible here. This is the time when health can still be maintained, even with only a modest effort. Regardless of the age of the health worshipers, if we could examine their psyche we would always find unresolved grief feelings. They are not willing or able to face their feelings of loss about their declining health. Instead they flee into idolatry, hoping that by idolizing health, they will never have to face their own finitude.

Idolization cannot endure, because health, like all false gods, is temporary, finite, and of "this world." In time one's health does decline, and then it becomes apparent to the once true believer that this god has failed. Idolatry fades in time. Perhaps it will be replaced with a new defense, or more likely, with despair. Or perhaps the former true believer will begin to deal with the feelings that he or she has ignored for so long. Then and only then is there an opportunity for that person to respond in faith and with realism.

This discussion of the idolatry of health raises several complex questions that cannot be addressed thoroughly in this chapter. One of the key questions is: Where is the line between a proactive health maintenance program and health worship? This is a very tricky question for every person who both cares about his or her health and who also wants to live in the way of faith. Unlike other losses of later life, the loss of health can be prevented or at least tempered with a proactive program of health maintenance. More and more people, especially people in the later years, are "health conscious" and are taking steps to keep themselves in good health. This is largely a positive development, one to rejoice in. From my perspective the key variable is whether a person has dealt realistically with his or her grief feelings. Persons who have worked through their grief feelings can embrace a health maintenance program and keep it in perspective. At the other extreme are persons who enter a health maintenance program, usually in an obsessive mode, as a way of avoiding their grief feelings. As Christians, we believe that the body is good and that God wants all people to live in full health as long as possible. However, health is not an end in itself; it is a means to an end. The end is always salvation. The person of faith will keep his or her sights set on the larger goal of life's journey and not get lured into worshiping health no matter how attractive that altar might appear.[4]

THE LOSS OF MAJOR BODY FUNCTIONS

As we continue to age into the sixth, seventh, and even eighth decades of life, the loss of health remains a constant theme. We must regularly deal with the little losses and declines that accompany each year. For many people, however, the next major time when the loss of health becomes a crucial issue occurs when they experience the loss of a major bodily function. The result of this loss is the first chronic condition or physical limitation. Examples of such losses would include the loss of sight, the loss of hearing, the loss of mobility, and the loss of sexual function. We not only have the loss per se to contend with, but now we must learn to live with some permanent physical limitation.

Our response to a major function loss is probably not going to be too dissimilar from our response to the earlier occasions of loss, except for two things. First, our response is more colored by fear than anger. By now the cumulative effect of loss upon loss has taken its toll on us. Death seems closer to us now than it used to be. We have less energy to fight back and more easily slip into despair, covered over by a veneer of disgust. The loss of a major body function also means the loss of independence, which we will discuss more specifically in the next chapter. This is a new wrinkle, a new challenge. This kind of loss of major bodily function is a frightening experience—particularly for people who have valued their independence and self-sufficiency.

The Academy Award-winning movie, *On Golden Pond,* was a wonderful study in aging, old age, and intergenerational healing. Henry Fonda and Katharine Hepburn played the principal roles with the richness and intensity of two great veterans of the theater. As the movie opens, Norman Thayer and his wife, Ethel, are coming to the summer cabin in late spring, next to Golden Pond, where apparently they had spent many previous summers. Now, however, Norman is approaching his eightieth birthday. He is struggling with his old age and declining health. His response is largely a not-too-subtle attitude of bitterness, sarcasm, and denial. He simultaneously knows that he has health limitations that he did not previously have, yet pretends that he can still work, fix doors, find directions, and drive motorboats the way he used to. Ethel's response is supportive and even upbeat, but also realistic.

In one particularly powerful scene, Ethel encourages Norman to pick strawberries down by the Old Town Road instead of looking for "gainful employment" in the newspaper's want ads. Grudgingly, Norm takes the pail and proceeds down the path. With a wonderful piece of acting and camera work, we then see Norman get disoriented and confused in the woods and then progressively more frightened. He does not recognize where he is and cannot find the Old Town Road. He becomes panicky. He is frightened and momentarily lost. Finally, in what probably seems like an eternity to Norman, he finds his way back to the cabin with an empty pail in hand and the perspiration of anxiety dripping from his face. He jokes his way through the awkward conversation with his wife and the mailman regarding why he returned so quickly and without any strawberries.

Later, when he and Ethel are alone, he reveals why he returned so quickly from the strawberry search in a dialogue that goes something like this:

> "You want to know why I came back so fast?" he says in a hostile tone. "I got to the end of our land and I couldn't remember where Old Town Road was. I wandered away there in the woods. Nothing looked familiar. It scared me half to death. . . . That's why I came back, to your pretty face, so I could feel safe, where I'm still me." In obvious anguish and humility, he then sits down, with his head in his hands.
>
> Ethel comforts him: "You're safe. You old fool. . . . Listen to me, Mister. You're my knight in shining armor. Don't you forget it. You're going to get back on that horse, me beside you, and away we go."
>
> "You're a pretty old dame, aren't you?" responds Norm. "What are you doing with an old dotty s.o.b. like me?"
>
> "I haven't the vaguest idea," she answers in obvious tones of grace and acceptance.

It's a wonderful scene. It portrays so well the terrible, frightening feeling of declining health and loss of function. The terror of the strawberry search reveals to us the intensity of Norman's anxiety that he normally covers over with sarcasm and disgust. The strawberry incident is clearly a concrete visualization of the larger, more pervasive struggle with old age that Norman Thayer is caught in. Feeling that we are losing our health evokes anxiety in all of us. Feelings of confusion, disorientation, anger, and panic lie just beneath the surface. It is all there in one scene—so particular and yet so universal.

CHRONIC HEALTH PROBLEMS

Some of the losses of health do not come upon us in major events. They come upon us as gradual processes. And in time they result in chronic health problems. Such losses in health, precisely because they are slow in developing, do not grab our attention. They are easy to ignore. They are easy to adjust to in little steps. But over time, as these declines in our health turn into chronic conditions, these changes wear on us and drain us of energy and optimism.

Chronic illness rises with age. It is reported that four out of five adults over sixty-five years old have at least one chronic condition and multiple conditions are common.[5] In a 1982 survey conducted by National Ambulatory Medical Care, the authors concluded that "chronic conditions are the most prevalent health problems" among the elderly, in contrast to the year 1900 when "acute conditions" were the predominant health problem for the elderly.[6] Today, the most prevalent chronic conditions among the elderly are: arthritis, hypertension disease, hearing impairments, and heart conditions. These conditions require long-term adjustment and adaptation.

Sometimes diseases become chronic and permanent precisely because we did not take them seriously enough sooner. Our denial got in our way. We ignored them. We were experiencing them as anxiety. We pushed their emergence into the back of our minds, as fearful reminders of our aging.

As with few other conditions, chronic health conditions wear on us. They drain us of energy and optimism. We can "rally" for a week or a year, but when such illnesses go on and on, year after year, we get discouraged. Our doctors and other caregivers become equally discouraged and frustrated. Most older adults with chronic conditions know the feeling that their doctors have "given up on them," because their condition can no longer be cured. To their doctors, they are "failures." Yet, this very frustration and this very "failure" mentality, confronts with the opportunity for a paradigm shift. It confronts us all with our overreliance upon a doing (and "curing") mode of valuing.

Henri J. M. Nouwen, who was mentioned in Chapter 7, has built upon the distinction between doing and being, which was helpful to our discussion of the loss of work, to make a parallel distinction between curing and caring.[7] The former is associated with Western culture's overemphasis upon doing; the latter virtue is associated with a being mode of valuing. Precisely because chronic health conditions cannot be cured, we are forced to think differently about our life, our values, and how to help others. Nouwen suggests that care and caring are the more appropriate and more important modes of valuing for the latter third of life. The chronic ailments of the elderly cannot be fixed. They cannot be cured; just as old age itself cannot be cured. Yet, in the midst of these conditions, we can learn to care, to adjust, to adapt, and to suffer with dignity and grace. This is the developmental task of the latter years, and in particular, during the repeated losses of health, to learn the art of suffering well, the virtue of "long suffering."

Nouwen does not stop there. He goes on to suggest that the elderly have a gift to give us, the nonelderly, those who would be caregivers to the elderly. Since we cannot fix them, or cure them, we too must learn the art of genuine caregiving. Nouwen writes:

> This is the great message of the elderly, not so much by what they say as by who they are. The elderly do not offer to the professional who is primarily concerned with cure much chance of satisfaction. They confront the doctor with the limitations of his healing powers, the psychologist with the relativity of self-fulfillment, the social worker with the lasting ambiguities in human relations, and the minister with the undeniable reality of death. In short, they confront all who live with the illusion of any final cure. But it is precisely this confrontation that opens the way for a constant reawakening of our primary call which is not to cure but to care.[8]

Nouwen goes on to say that genuine caring is listening, is learning "to be with" and is an openness to our own vulnerability. This is the gift that the elderly can give us, we who interact with, work with, and love older adults, to value caring over curing. Often what the older person wants most and finds most helpful, is genuine caring, and in this culture that overemphasizes doing, that is the quality that we have least of and are least well trained in. This is our opportunity to learn caring, the developmental task of this phase of life characterized by chronic losses of health.

TRANSCENDING THE BODY

The spiritual challenge that awaits us all as our health declines from minor losses to major limitations and chronic conditions is to increasingly transcend the body. This is not an easy assignment. We are accustomed to equating ourselves with our bodies. If my body is sick, I say, "I'm sick." Or if my body is well today, I say, "I feel fine today." We are not accustomed to separating ourselves from our bodies. We are naturally wholistic. Yet many older people, especially spiritually sensitive people, tell me that as they get older they are able to distinguish themselves more and more from their bodies. They begin to realize that their essence, their true being, is not limited to their physical condition. They realize that their mind, their spirit, and their personality can be still very healthy and very alive, even while their body is declining in vigor. We might even say that such people have discovered their souls. By shifting perspectives on themselves in this way, they are able to increasingly transcend the body's limitations.

Obviously this kind of spiritual maturity is rare among the general population. Most people do not seem to rise above their ailments, except on momentary occasions. It is hard to transcend the body. In fact, many older people develop what Robert C. Peck calls "body preoccupation."[9] They become increasingly absorbed with their bodies and its subtle aches, pains, and changes. We have all met older people who seem to talk endlessly about their last surgery or who can describe in detail yesterday's bowel movement or who despair at length about their declining strength. Obviously the bodily hurts and our physical limitations can cause us great pain and frustration. It is difficult to transcend pain. It is easy to become absorbed with one's body over the passing years.

If you recall the rest of that movie, *On Golden Pond*, you will remember that Norman's daughter (played by Jane Fonda) leaves her thirteen-year-old stepson-to-be with Norm and Ethel for a month, while she and his father travel elsewhere. As the story unfolds, we see the interplay between generations, young adolescent and old man. By the time the movie ends, Norman is no longer the bitter, despairing old man that he was at the start of the summer. In my terminology, Norman has momentarily "transcended his body" and begun to focus on the things of the spirit: relationships, sharing, enjoying, and being. It is a powerful argument for the value of intergenerational contact and relationships. He experiences again that the real Norman is not his body, but his spirit.

Learning to suffer well or transcend the body is not easy.[10] It does require a very subtle but important change in our self-understanding. We need to see ourselves more and more as spiritual beings, not as earthly creatures. Our bodies, like all things of "this world" are finite, temporary, and fragile. Our real worth lies in our spirits, our souls, our personalities. To put it in different terms, most of our lives we have valued *doing* modes—producing, accomplishing, making, having. Now, we need to come to value *being* modes—understanding, sharing, knowing.[11] For most of our lives we have valued ourselves and been valued for what we produced, how we looked, what we owned, or what we earned. Now God's challenge to us in our old age is to shift modes of valuing from having to being. If we do so, we can learn to value ourselves for who we are. We can increasingly learn to nurture our souls even while our bodies are declining.

THE VALUE OF BEING HANDICAPPED

Everyone should know at least one handicapped person. Charlotte was crippled in an automobile accident at age seventeen, and has been on crutches ever since. I have had the privilege to walk (literally and figuratively) with Charlotte for many years as her friend and counselor and pastor. I have listened to her despair at being "deformed" and her frustration at being helpless. I have listened to her anger at how "people stare at my legs, not because they're pretty, but because I'm a freak or something." I have grieved for her for the life that might have been. I have listened to her questions about whether she would ever marry or could ever hope to cope with children. Yet I have also admired her courage as she pushed her limits again and again. I have been instructed by her humility and gratitude toward what health she does have. And I have seen what a genuinely beautiful, spiritual person she has become over the years.

There is a handicapped person in your future—you! Handicapped persons are dealing in the present moment with what you and I will have to deal with later. Sooner or later, each of us will become handicapped in one way or another. Sooner or later, each of us will have to deal with one or several major losses in our health. Then we will travel down the same path as handicapped persons. Then we will know their pain, frustration, and sufferings. Perhaps if we could learn from them now, whatever our age, we would be better prepared for our own future.

Handicapped persons teach us that life is more than a body. They demonstrate the truth of all great religions: that the qualities that make us truly human and truly divine are not physical. They are qualities of the Spirit. St. Paul listed a few of these qualities: love, joy, peace, patience, kindness, goodness, faithfulness, gentleness, self-control (Gal 5:22). Jesus listed a few more: meekness, peacemaking, purity of heart, mercy, hunger for righteousness, suffering in a right cause (Mt 5:3-10). Neither of them mentioned physical beauty or even physical health. The qualities that save us do not include bodily health and beauty.

Handicapped persons also can teach us how to suffer and how to rise above bodily limitations. Sometimes pain cannot be fixed, nor can all limitations be conquered. Most of us will have to deal with pain and limitations, at first in minor ways and later in major ways. We will learn new meanings for "courage." Either we will rise above our limitations and learn to live with them, or we will sink to new lows of despair, bitterness, and helplessness. The choice depends largely on the depth of our courage.

In a sense, then, a handicap or a loss of health can become a gift. It never starts out that way. Initially it is a horrible loss. If through the loss, however, we can learn to nurture our spiritual qualities and learn the art of suffering well, then we will have transformed our loss into gain. We will have grown in and through our loss. We will have risen above our loss precisely by not letting it defeat us, but by letting it propel us into a more advanced stage of human existence. Admittedly, not everyone makes such a major leap forward. Neither have some human beings made it past a Sunday school theology. Yet, the loss of health in later life, as horrible as it seems, can be the opportunity for growth in spiritual maturity.

Chapter 9

The Loss of Independence

My grace is sufficient for you, for my power is made perfect in weakness.

II Cor 12:9

We cannot escape the gradual loss of independence that comes with each decline in our health. When a person loses a major physical function, such as sight, hearing, or mobility, the dependency becomes very obvious and very real. Now we are "impaired," "handicapped" . . . and we must deal with the assorted feelings that go with those labels. We must deal with the loss of independence, the loss of self-reliance, the loss of control, and the corresponding diminishing of self-worth that these losses imply in this culture.

Yet, the loss of independence is broader and more pervasive than those losses associated with declines in our health. The loss of independence is implied in the loss of a home, the loss of mobility, and the decline of income—all of which occur in the second half of life. The loss of independence can begin in retirement for people who do not have adequate retirement income. Financial restrictions limit personal freedom and their range of choices. The loss of independence can be experienced again when one's spouse dies. In the aftermath of that loss, we become aware of how dependent we had become on him or her. Now, to age well, we have to learn to be more self-reliant and practice greater independence.

If old age is entering our "second childhood," as some writers have termed it, then the dynamics of independence and dependency are pervasive; only this time, we experience not the gradual gaining of independence, but the gradual losing of independence. So if we are to age well through these years, we must grieve this loss in graceful and mature ways. Grieving our loss of independence includes becoming comfortable with our growing dependency . . . but not too comfortable. In a strange sort of way the very "letting go" of our need for independence can free us for a new and fresh appreciating and embracing of the remaining independence we do have available to us in our later years.

LOSS OF HOME

Most of us who live in urban or suburban areas do not easily appreciate the deep roots that some people can attach to their home and to the land. In smaller communities or in rural communities, it is not uncommon for several generations of a family to have been born and raised in the same home or on the same land. People say "that's the Taylor house" or "the Wheeler farm," because some Taylor or some Wheeler has lived on that land for as long as anyone can remember.

When a person grows old, however, and the spouse is dead, and the children have moved away, and then health fades, there comes a time when he or she may have to move out of the cherished family home. Usually this "final" relocation is into a health care facility or an adult child's home where the older adult can be cared for more fully and lovingly. The loss of home or homestead can be a difficult loss for many. People often have deep emotional attachments to their home.

Ethel was one such person. Her pastor told me about Ethel and the difficulty she experienced in moving from her home of forty-seven years. She and her husband built the home when they were "young kids" fresh out of high school. They planted the back acre and added a room later when the family grew bigger. Altogether, they raised five children in their home. In recent years, Ethel has lived alone in the big house, which is somewhat distant from town. She has fallen several times, and her growing arthritis was making it difficult for her to care for herself. Her daughter, Karen, felt strongly that it was time for her mother to move into her home in St. Louis where they could easily add a bedroom or rent her a nearby apartment. There was just one problem—Ethel didn't want to move. The pastor who was involved in trying to talk to Ethel remembers some of the conversation.

"This is my home. Charles and I built this place. I know every nook and cranny. I have painted each wall a dozen times. The stain over there on the rug is from when Jack was sick as a baby, and those marks on the wall are from measuring the children's heights, and the apple tree out back was put in when our Inky (their family dog) died. It's all here, pastor, my whole life. I feel at home here. This is where I belong, not in some small noisy apartment in a city.

"You have a lot of memories here—wonderful memories. It's a hard place to leave," the pastor responded.

"What would happen to me there? It wouldn't be the same."

"Oh, you wouldn't be the same?" he inquired, "Is that what you fear? You know, you really wouldn't stop being yourself. You'll take that with you—the memories, the furniture, the pictures, your faith."

"You're so kind, Pastor," she said as only a woman in her eighth decade can say to a minister half her age. "It's hard to leave behind all of this. It's so much a part of me."

"You know, the Lord God asked Abraham to get up and leave his home one time and he wasn't much older than you. God didn't even tell him where he was going, only that he had to go and that He would go with him. I have often thought of how frightening that must have been for Abraham. . . ."

"Did Abraham go?"

"Yes, Abraham went," the pastor continued, smiling. "He went because he knew that where he was was not as important as whom he was with. You might say that he was a pilgrim, moving from place to place, never settling too long at any one place, lest he forget that his ultimate home is beyond this world."

"I guess God wants me to be a pilgrim too—but I don't like it much."

The pastor reported to me that Ethel did go to live with her daughter and still later to a "home" for the aged. It was not an easy transition for her, but the image of the pilgrim seemed to help some. "It's a good image," remarked the pastor. "After all, we are all pilgrims in this life and periodically we must pick up and go."

What is clear from this example is that moving out of a long-time home is more than the mere loss of a house. It is also a loss of independence. It means that we cannot take care of ourselves any longer. We are becoming more dependent, more helpless, more passive . . . less self-reliant. It is the marker event that crystallizes this loss of independence.

RESIDENTIAL CHANGES
AS A FUNCTION OF INDEPENDENCE

The initial change or loss of residence, as described in Ethel's story, is not an easy change to make and is often experienced as the "marker event" that symbolizes our loss of independence. Yet, it may not be our last change of residence. Throughout the last third of the life cycle, an older adult's residence is often determined by his or her relative health and corresponding relative degree of self-reliance.

Bernice L. Neugarten, one of the leading gerontologists of our time, has categorized the "new" old age into three parts: "the young old," "the old," and "the old old."[1] This distinction is based on the degrees of a person's relative autonomy rather than on chronology. People who can still live independently, who can still maintain an active life, perhaps working part-time and who need but routine medical care, fall into the category of the "young old." The "old" need semi-independent living situations, where some routine support functions, such as meal preparation, are provided and where medical care is easily available. The third category of people, "the old old," must have full-time medical care and are largely unable to live independently due to their health limitations. These "stages" are not always neatly divided. Some people might go back and forth between several stages before transitioning to the next phase of residential care.

Each of these changes in the relative independence of a person's living situation may involve a change in residence. Many homes or residential communities for the aged cater to one level of need or another. Thus, they may require that the resident move on when he or she has passed onto another level of need. For many people the most desirable living situations are those residential communities that have all three levels of care available on the same campus. This arrangement allows people to pass easily from one level of care to another with the least disruption in their lives, and if necessary this arrangement also allows them to alternate between levels of care. The general rule of thumb here is to try to maintain the most independence possible for an individual without endangering his or her health. Caregivers know that a sense of independence, however relative it might be, does much to help a person maintain a positive attitude toward life.

When dealing with this difficult subject of declining independence and residential location or relocation, there is no substitute for advanced planning. The more we can anticipate our future health limitations and make plans accordingly, the easier time we will have with these transitions when they arrive. Planning ahead is possible only if we have dealt with our feelings about our present and future losses in health. If we deny those inevitable changes, we will avoid making plans and probably, when the time comes for a necessary relocation, the decision will be made for us rather than by us.

Florence was one of the wise, forward-planning people. When she was in her sixties and still in fairly good health, she lived alone in an apartment complex for senior citizens. It was a nice apartment in a very pleasant location. There was no reason to move, but one day she put her name in for the new Senior Citizen Towers that was being constructed down the block, "Why?" I asked her. "Why would you want to leave this nice cozy place?"

"The stairs," she noted. "I won't always be able to get up those stairs when I get older. I need to get into a place that has elevators. And I'll want a smaller place then, one that I can manage easily."

She was anticipating the loss of health that was to come. She had been around old people often enough so that she knew what was ahead of her—and she was right. She did become less mobile over the years that followed. Her bad foot became more and more difficult to walk on, but long before that happened, she had moved into an efficiency apartment in the new Senior Citizen Towers where she did not have to contend with stairs. She was one person who not only accepted the reality of declining health, but actually planned for it in a realistic way. Her response was not denial or despair, but a realistic appraisal of her future and appropriate action. She prepared herself and thus she was able to make her loss of health a nonproblem. She passed through the transition from independent to semi-independent living with ease. She was able to spend her time and energy on more important matters during those years than on worrying about how she was going to negotiate the stairs each day.

LOSS OF MOBILITY

Another "marker event" that often symbolizes or crystallizes the loss of independence is the "giving up" or loss of one's driver's license, an event that usually occurs in the later decades of life.

Driving an automobile has always been equated with independence. That is what driving an automobile meant when we were teenagers. We could not wait for the privilege. Being mobile afforded us great independence. We did not have to ask Dad or Mom to take us somewhere. So too in old age, driving still is equated with independence. Seniors that are still driving can get themselves to the market, to the doctor, to church. . . . and at their own schedule. For adults that have driven all of their lives and are used to that mobility, convenience, and independence, the loss of their driver's license is a big change in their lifestyle . . . perhaps a dramatic loss. The loss of one's driver's license is a powerful symbol that announces to ourselves (and to the world) that we are now homebound, that we are helpless and/or that we are truly "old."

The very week I was writing this chapter, Ruth came to see me for her monthly "checkup" counseling session. Ruth is a seventy-five-year-old senior, who has always cherished her independence. Since she was thirty-five years old, after an unwelcome divorce, she repeatedly reminds me, she has worked for a living and supported herself. When her health and people skills faded in the last five years, she reduced her hours to part time . . . but work, yes, she always has worked right up through the present day.

"I'm in trouble with the DMV (Department of Motor Vehicles), right up to my ear lobes," was her opening statement at our counseling session.

When she had gone in to renew her driver's license, she passed the written test well enough and the eye test, but as she was writing out the check to pay the renewal fees, her hand trembled, as it usually did the last few years, making her handwriting illegible. Noticing, the clerk put her renewal forms aside.

"They gave me a sixty-day permit and scheduled a hearing in June to review the matter. I have to get my doctor to fill out these forms . . . if I only hadn't written that check. Maybe my doctor can give me a pill or something."

"I don't recall what your driving record is like," I stated.

"You're right. My record is clean. I think I would know it if I couldn't drive, if I was a risk."

"Maybe they don't want you to have even that first accident," I observed.

"You know, it never entered my mind that there might come a time when I couldn't drive for physical reasons. I considered that I might not be able to afford a car some time, but not this. This has been a shock. Maybe by this time next month, I won't be able to drive. Do you make house calls, Doctor?"

"I guess I'll have to start considering such," I responded. "Think some more about how your life might change."

"You mean, if I'm grounded. . . . I guess I would have to take Dial-A-Ride or something, like the rest of the old folks. You know how impatient I am. That will kill me, waiting for that stupid bus half the day. And, oh yes, my volunteer work which I just love. . . . that will be just too far to get to.

"'Grounded' is a good word for it." I noted. "This will be a severe limiting of your freedom."

"You know me, Doc," asserting her independence. "If I have to lose my driver's license, I'll fight it all the way."

For Ruth and for most older adults, the loss of mobility, particularly as it is expressed in the loss of a driver's license, is related to a decline in health. In 1990, there were 33 million citizens age sixty-five or over. Of that number, approximately 24.7 million held valid drivers' licenses—nearly two-thirds of them under the age of seventy-five years.[2] The number of older adults with drivers licenses falls off dramatically in the seventh and eighth decades of life. The loss of one's driver's license, either voluntarily or involuntarily, is an inevitable part of the late life-adjustments.

Since the loss of one's driver's license carries such practical and symbolic importance, it is easy for the issue to get caught up in the same dynamics as the loss of health discussed in the last chapter. If a man is denying his declining independence and hates the thought of being dependent, he may insist on driving well beyond a time when it is safe to do so. Or if a woman is rationalizing away her poor eyesight, she will rationalize the decline of her driving skills too. The feelings of denial, anger, and rationalization can get acted out behind the wheel, which can be a very dangerous place to do one's grief work.[3]

CLINGING TO LOST INDEPENDENCE

Independence consists of our ability to live life as we choose, to be self-directed and competent. It is a sense of personal power. It is one of our most prized possessions. We struggle for it at age four and five. We demand it at age fourteen and eighteen. Now in our later years we watch it slip through our grasp like sand through the hourglass. We resent it. We try to hide it. We cling to it . . . sometimes in artificial and sometimes in realistic ways.

It is difficult to give up independence. In aging we often don't have a choice, we can only accept it or not accept it, grieve it or cling to what is lost. Clinging to a lost independence, or in the terminology of this book, making an idol out of what is lost, can be dangerous:

- Resisting the loss of independence may mean continuing to drive a car well beyond the time that it is safe to do so.
- Denying health limitations, a person may still insist on climbing up on the roof of the house to clean the rain gutters—an activity that is now quite risky.
- A woman may refuse to use a cane or a wheelchair and thereby run the risk of a fall that would injure her still further.
- A man may refuse to wear his hearing aid . . . "it makes him look old" . . . and run a risk of not hearing a siren or even his boss.
- A woman may insist on continuing to live alone in the family home, even after she has fallen twice and left the burner on all night once—both considerable risks.
- A man may refuse to ask his children for financial help, and try to make ends meet by turning off the heat at night, an unwise if not risky decision.

I am sure that these examples and many others that come to mind, serve to illustrate that: clinging to lost independence can be dangerous.

LOSS OF FINANCIAL SECURITY

The loss of income can also mean a loss of independence. Most older adults enter the last third of life with a loss of income. Usually that decline in income occurs around retirement, in which the older adult goes from receiving a full-time income to a partial income or income derived from Social Security and pension sources. The loss of income is certainly part of the loss of work experience, but it is noted here as part of the loss of independence as well. In addition, older Americans also may experience another decline of income when their spouse dies, and perhaps another associated with a major loss of health.

Many older adults have substantially less cash income than those under sixty-five years. In 1984, for example, the median family income of a head of family sixty-five or older was less than two-thirds of the median income of a head of family between the ages of twenty-five and sixty-four.[4] Since then there have been some encouraging signs as a result of Social Security increases and other factors. Yet these improvements are deceiving, because the conclusions are generalized for all older people. And some older adults live with a severely reduced income. A 1987 study, funded by the Commonwealth Fund, argued that older people with the greatest risk of sinking below the poverty level are widows and persons with significant health-related expenses due to a dramatic decline of their health—two typical developmental losses discussed earlier in this book.[5]

This overall reduction in financial resources,and the potential decline of financial resources associated with two typical losses in later life, translates into a loss of independence. This loss or change will affect people differently. For most older adults, this means not buying what they wish, or going where they wish, or living the lifestyle they might wish. It may result in having to rely on adult children for supplemental income. And/or it may means that the senior cannot live independently at all and may have to live with his or her adult children. Such dependece is difficult and most older adults resist it. Most do not wish to be "a bother" to their adult children.

LOSS OF CONTROL

The loss of independence is, among other things, a loss of control or personal power. Further, dependency is feared in large measure because it embodies a fear of being controlled by others or victimized by events beyony our control.

The issue of control is one of those psychological problems that bothers many people, young and old alike.[6] The issue is captured nicely in the lines from the Serenity Prayer: "God grant me the serenity to accept the things I cannot change; courage to change the things I can; and the wisdom to know the difference."[7] It is the latter phrase that seems to trip up many people. How do we know if a particular situation is something we can control or something that we must accept with serenity?

Life's difficulties run the broad spectrum between being 100 percent out of our control, (an earthquake), or being 100 percent within our control, (our driving record). Few events are pure. Most events have some elements that are within our control and some elements that are beyond our control. Thus, we can have trouble determining whether we should assert ourselves, fight back, and try to mediate or change the course of events, or whether we should passively accept these circumstances as "God's will" and strive to be at peace with our fate. Out of this confusion we may try to control things we cannot control or accept with resignation some things that we should try to control.

This issue can be applied to the psychology of the later years of life. As we pass through these various losses, changes, and transitions, how do we know how to respond? Do we try to resist these losses and run the risk of raising denial to a new art form? Or do we accept these losses with as much grace and serenity as we can? In this book, I have certainly advocated for the importance of recognizing and grieving the losses of later life, and yet the situation is often more complicated when it comes to the loss of independence.

The concept of "learned helplessness" offers some interesting insights into this issue.[8] Researchers experimenting with rats which were being randomly shocked discovered that if the rat had some measure of control over the frequency and intensity of the shocks, the rat handled the trauma. Whereas if the rat had no control over the shocks' frequency or intensity, the rat "gave up," became apathetic . . . and some time later, even when the circumstances had changed and the rat now had the ability to alleviate the situation, the rat remained in the state of "learned helplessness." Psychologists have described this learned helplessness as depression or despair.

Similarly, it has been demonstrated that when humans are subjected to a series of painful and traumatic events, they can cope with these horrible events if they perceive that they have some measure of control or choice, however small or large, over the what is happening. Conversely, humans who experience traumatic events as random, unpredictable, and out of their control, become apathetic, despairing, or as someone who has learned to be helpless.

I believe that many older adults experience life in the later years in exactly this way—as a series of traumatic losses that seem to be out of their control. Having been so beaten down or "made" helpless, they resign themselves to a kind of chronic despair, just waiting for the next wave of illness, loss, or death itself.

Some additional relevant data on the dynamics of control surround the concept of "locus of control."[9] Researchers here distinguish between those persons who perceive themselves to have an internal locus of control and those individuals who perceive an external locus of control. Testing instruments can determine an individual's dominant perception: internal or external locus of control. Individuals who largely see events as controlled by external forces or factors, see those events as beyond their control. They see themselves as pawns on the board game of life. In contrast, individuals who favor an internal locus of control, tend to see events or situations as controllable by themselves. People who favor an internal locus of control tend to take the initiative, look for ways to improve their situation, and act in pro-active ways. One's perception of locus of control, in reference to an unfolding unwelcomed event, will determine how actively or passively that person responds to those events.

Both of these bodies of research[10]—the material on learned helplessness and the material on locus of control—suggest to us that older adults can handle losses well if they perceive themselves as having some measure of control or influence over the events. They can act, not just react. They can impact or shape events, not just have things happen to them. Some losses in later life, especially the unexpected ones, can be pretty overwhelming. Yet, any measure of control or choice, however small, will go a long way to empower the individual and mobilize his or her coping mechanisms and health resources. Or to use the language of independence and dependence, when an older adult gives in to dependency as a mind-set, he or she has learned helplessness. Chronic dependency leads to apathy, despair, and rapid aging.[11] A sense of independence or personal control empowers the individual, and helps one feel young.

This insight has many applications. The principle is being applied more and more to work with the sick, the aged, and those otherwise traumatized. Nurses tell us that patients who are able to control the administration of their own pain medicine often do better, not because the medicine is better, but because they are in control. They are being empowered. Doctors often want post-surgical patients to get up and get moving as soon as possible. Besides being physically better, they want such patients to avoid "giving in" to feeling dependent. Researchers tell us that people in nursing homes improve remarkably after altering their lives, sometimes in "the simplest ways—giving them a potted plant to tend, allowing them to make up their own menus and take charge of tidying their rooms. Instead of being passive, lonely dependents, playing the role of 'old folks in a nursing home,' these people regained a sense of usefulness and worth."[12]

Wherever possible give older adults a choice. Wherever possible teach older adults to do it themselves, instead of doing it "to them" or "for them." Wherever possible, help older adults to exercise some control, however small. Wherever and whenever possible, we should allow for and facilitate individuals' independence, while adjusting to their growing dependency. Above all else, treat older adults with dignity and respect.[13]

We know that seniors become more dependent in the later years. That's a fact. It cannot be avoided. On one hand we must grieve this loss, let go of our lost independence. Yet, on the other hand, we must look for ways to encourage what independence is still possible. We know from this research that a sense of independence or control is a health enhancer and a health mobilizer.

A CULTURE OF INDEPENDENCE

We live in a culture that prizes independence, even idolizes independence. We live in a culture that also prizes the individual—the individual's rights, the individual's worth, and the individual's freedom. In this cultural context, dependency has taken on negative connotations. We do not like people who are overly dependent. We do not like having to take care of people who are overly dependent, be they sick, or on welfare, or handicapped. We certainly do not like it when we, for whatever reason, become dependent. We would prefer to be self-reliant. We would prefer that we were a nation of "rugged individualists."

Yet, we must also state the obvious: people become more dependent as they enter the last third of their lives and especially after major declines in their health. This dependency is multifaceted. It includes physical dependency, as in needing help to maintain a house and prepare meals. It includes financial dependency, as in needing extra income each month. It includes psychological dependency, as in needing the support of others.

I believe that one of the reasons why we, as a culture, tend to isolate and shun the elderly is that we do not like their dependency. We equate dependency with low self-worth, and independence with high self-worth. We find their dependency repulsive . . . maybe even frightening. We would rather pay someone else to take care of Grandfather or Aunt Susan. We would rather not see them or be burdened with their needs. In short, the way we choose to treat the elderly in this culture is a reflection of America's overemphasis on independence, autonomy, and individualism. Thus, we tend to ill-prepare ourselves and our loved ones for the inevitable dependency that comes with age.

If we tend to equate dependency with low self-worth and independence, or autonomy, with high self-worth, how do we suppose elderly people in this culture feel about themselves when they become more dependent? Perhaps they tend to feel embarrassed, shamed, unwilling to acknowledge or admit it. Would it be easy or difficult to accept one's growing loss of independence? Would it be easy or difficult to ask for help?

The trick to aging well is to enable older persons to let go of their lost independence without feeling a corresponding loss of self-worth. The goal is to help older or handicapped people to befriend their dependency without feeling diminished in value and respect.

LETTING GO, TO RECEIVE

Speaking as a psychologist, I would like to point out that independence and dependence are relative terms. They are not right or wrong, or good or bad. What one culture or even one individual considers "dependent" may be perceived or experienced by another as "an autonomous act." Further, each of us is a mixture of independent and dependent traits. Each of us has needs in both areas. No one is pure independence or always 100 percent dependent.[14] The healthy person will have some elements of both. At times and in certain roles we need to feel strong, independent, and self-reliant. At other times or in other roles, we also need to feel close to others, secure with others, and as one who belongs in community. How each of us blends our needs for independence and dependence and how we choose to manifest those needs, will vary widely from individual to individual. The key to good mental health and effective interpersonal functioning is learning to recognize and balance our relative needs, knowing when to be independent and when to be dependent, and the ability to be comfortable in either mode. Or to phrase it still differently, we need to befriend dependency, without internalizing the diminished self-esteem that this culture places on dependency.

Sometimes if we look at a situation objectively, giving up our denials and cultural expectations, letting go of our vain attempts to cling to independence and acknowledge our growing dependency, we will be able to make adjustments that might just allow us to maintain more independence than we might otherwise believe possible.

Ruth, who we met earlier in this chapter, fought fiercely to retain her drivers license. Unfortunately, it was a losing battle. She did not give up this loss of independence easily. The years that followed were difficult ones of declining wellness. With each passing month and year, she became more and more isolated and lonely. She rarely went out of the house. She stopped her volunteer work. She hated her life, and especially her lack of freedom and independence. For her, being dependent was equated with death.

About two years later, someone persuaded her to relocate to a senior citizen housing complex. There she was able to access the free "shuttle" for transportation. She began to go places again. She was able to get out of her apartment much more often than she had, not only for trips, but even for walks about the grounds which were safer compared to where she had been living. Further, she was not as lonely as before. There were friends and planned activities several times a week that gave Ruth occasions to socialize. Her conclusion, when I spoke with her by phone sometime later, was that "I'm more independent now than I was before. Why didn't you tell me about this place sooner?"

Ruth's transition illustrates the paradox of independence and dependence in the later years. By letting go of her lost independence, or to paraphrase, by embracing her dependency, Ruth was able to make adjustments and actually realize a measure of independence which she would not have otherwise thought possible. This would not have been possible if she had not grieved her loss of independence experienced in the loss of her automobile. If she had continued to cling to that lost illusion, she would have never realized the independence that was still possible for her at this stage of life.

Newly handicapped people (and remember we are all going to be handicapped some day) go through a similar process. They must grieve the loss of wholeness and come to terms with their anger, sorrow, and limitations. They must, in a sense, befriend their dependency, while at the same time, not internalizing any diminished value because they are dependent. They must continue to maintain an internal locus of control, not take on the attitude of a victim, and then and only then, will they begin to mobilize what resources they do have available, fight back in areas that can be influenced, and earn a measure of independence not otherwise possible. It is a strange paradox, a delicate balance—giving up control to gain some control, grieving lost independence in order to have the resources to reclaim independence.

THE VALUE OF SURRENDER

The loss of independence, like all of the losses of the later years, can be experienced both as event and process. The loss of independence can start around midlife in several subtle ways, but the central focus of this loss occurs more in the last third to last quarter of our life cycle, when the decline in our health has such a devastating effect. Some of us will not live to experience this stage of life. Many others, especially women, will struggle with the twin losses of health and independence that dominate this phase of our earthly journeys. These are not easy years. It is hard to see what good can emerge from them. It is hard to see what spiritual insights or growth can arise from these struggles. And yet, I believe that every stage of life has its lessons and its potential for deepening our "Christian walk."

The loss of independence certainly can teach us the value of surrender. The Christian faith has always placed great importance on this value. Our spiritual journey begins only when we surrender our wills, our hearts, and our lives to the Almighty God. We strive as humans, sometimes in absurd and vain ways, to maintain the illusion of self-sufficiency and independence. Yet ultimately, none of us is an island. We need other people and they need us. We need God and in a sense God needs us. Life is not an island, but a fabric of interwoven relationships. The psychological wars over dependence and independence need to be transcended by the ideal of interdependence, which is closer to the reality of human existence and closer to the Creator's desire for humanity.

The secret to a healthy life in the later years is found, in the words of the Serenity Prayer, "the wisdom to know the difference." "Wisdom" is a virtue born in the later years. It comes from a merging of knowledge and experience. It is a crown worn by the aged, or those who have lived long enough and suffered long enough, to know "the difference" . . . between when to be courageous and when to surrender, when to be independent and when to be dependent, and when to maintain control and when to give it up. And embedded in that wisdom is a spiritual mystery that surrendering is sometimes the path to control, that dependency is sometimes the path to independence, and that grieving is sometimes the path to new life. In the growing loss of independence, we have the opportunity to learn the truth of this mystery, and so prepare ourselves for the final transition.

Chapter 10

Faith and Successful Aging

For whoever would save his life will lose it, and whoever loses his life for my sake will find it.

Mt 16:25

We have completed our survey of the major losses in the later years of life. We have described some of the unique features of each loss. As was noted at the start of this book, these losses have not been presented in any chronological order. In fact, these losses are as much themes in later life as they are specific loss events. They are both events and processes. The loss of parents, for example, while associated with a specific event, can also be experienced as process as they decline in vitality. Further, the loss of health or the loss of youth are experienced primarily as processes, but even here specific marker events crystallize our awareness of the loss.

Given the pervasive presence and power of losses in later life, we now ask the question in this final chapter: How can we age well? Why do some people cope easily with the losses of later life while others seem to deteriorate mentally, spiritually, and physically? What are the ingredients that enable one to age well? Put on your theological caps and think for a moment about the nature of life in the later years, about human faith, and about God's grace in our lives.

THE FINAL LOSS

One major loss in later life has not been directly discussed, that is, the loss of our own life. I have chosen not to deal with our own death as a loss for several reasons. Chiefly, our own death is not a developmental loss in the normal sense of the word. Our own death is not a loss that we experience after the fact—at least not in this life. Its influence on our lives is entirely anticipatory.

In another sense, of course, our personal demise is *the ultimate loss*. It is the loss that stands behind—or, should I say, ahead of—all other losses. It is the loss that colors and influences every other loss. It is the loss that makes all of us anxious, an anxiety that becomes the very background music to life itself. In a sense we do live through this loss every time we lose anyone or anything we love.

Some people have suggested that the fear of death is really a young person's problem. People who live many years do not fear death as much as people in the prime of life. As death comes close, many people make peace with "the enemy." They anticipate it. They do their grief work in advance, and in many cases, especially when physical pain has been severe, death comes as a relief, as a welcome friend. I am not convinced that this adage is universally true. Yet it is true enough that it should give us cause to reflect on its dynamic.

One of the reasons why death is not always feared as much among the old as it is among the young is because most older people have lived through many small deaths. Death is nothing new to them. Hopefully, they also have experienced many resurrections. Perhaps they have discovered that new life does emerge out of the ashes of the old. If they have been fortunate enough to experience this dying and rising process once, even several times, then they are prepared for their ultimate trial. Such people can and do approach their own deaths with a kind of experiential confidence.

Mabel was an eighty-three-year-old retired Christian missionary with whom I had a delightful conversation about her life and approaching death. She often told me in her later years that she did not fear death, but neither did she boast of such assurance as many Christians do. Her attitude toward her own death was just a quiet confidence that fascinated me greatly. On one occasion I pursued the theme with her.

"Death has become my friend," she remarked, "an ever-present companion in my old age. I guess you get used to it—death. I don't fear it as much as I used to. It will come to me in good time, no sooner, no later."

"What has enabled you to overcome the fear?" I asked.

"I don't know that I have entirely. It's still alarming when I get sick. But I think I now fear the pain of dying more than death itself . . . I have more faith in God than I used to. Isn't it really a fear of the unknown? Isn't that all it is—just the unknown? If so, then I have faced the unknown before, many times."

"Describe for me one of those times when you faced the unknown," I continued.

"The one that I recall most was when Christopher and I first went out to the mission field. That was a real unknown! We didn't have any idea of what was going to happen to us; we just knew that this was something we had to do. I was pregnant at the time with Martha, and Timothy was three years old. Surely, part of me didn't want to leave our church in Maryland. It was comfortable. It was a fine congregation. We were surrounded by many loving people there."

"They were not easy years," she continued, "those years in the mission field. . . . Not easy at all. One time Chris got sick with malaria, and there I was in a strange country with two young children, no means of support, and a sick, possibly dying husband."

"Those were your darkest hours?" I asked. "What did you do?"

"I don't remember exactly. I think I just sat down and cried. It's funny, though, because now when I look back on those years, I think of them as the very best years of our lives. We made wonderful friends during that time, people who still call us and write us. Last year one of the young girls from one of our mission families came to this country for college. She stopped to see us. Too bad Christopher was not here anymore to see her. She is so grown up, so mature."

"New life came out of a situation that initially you thought would be a disaster," I observed.

"I guess that's why I don't fear death as much. God stayed with Chris and me during those times, and they turned into the best of times. I really believe that 'In all things God works for good for those who love him.' I know this to be true in my life, and that's what takes the edge off of death for me. . . . But those were rough times."

"God transformed your darkness into light, your worst times into the best times, your death into new life."

"Yes, indeed," she concluded.

Many of the transitions of life, like that of Mabel's relocation to the mission field, involve mini-death experiences. In this case it was the

death of a lifestyle in Maryland. In other situations a home is left behind, or someone may have died —a spouse or a parent. In other cases
a role has died. We are no longer a parent or a son or a daughter or an
executive. In almost all cases some part of us, some piece of our worth
or identity, has died. Maybe our sense of self-worth has been diminished because we no longer work. Maybe our good health has van-
ished. Perhaps our appearance has faded. Each and every loss event
described in this book carries with it a type of death, and every death
brings with it grief and sorrow.

We need to grieve these many "deaths" if we expect to pass
through to new life. We cannot hold back or get sidetracked in idolatry.
We must enter fully into our pain and suffering. We must also enter the
fear—the fear of the unknown future, as Mabel put it—that comes
with every transition. If we grieve well, then in time we do come to the
other side of sorrow. We do recapture our emotional energies and
begin again to invest ourselves into new loves, new identities, new
attachments. In the process of doing all this, we discover something
very amazing. We discover that we are different than we were before
the loss. We are now new persons. We have been changed, even
transformed, by the very process of grieving itself. We have passed
over into a new stage of our lives and with that passage we have taken
on a new role, a new identity, new priorities, and new relationships.
New life has emerged out of loss.

So grief has a history. How we have handled the various developmental losses in our lives influences how we shall handle the loss
currently before us, even if that loss is the loss of our own life. If we
have successfully grieved earlier losses, then the psychological pattern
is set.[1] We approach the current loss with confidence and trust. If we
have not grieved well, and remain stuck in varying degrees of idolatry,
then we find the current approaching loss to be terrorizing and paralyz-
ing. So faith has a developmental history that prepares us (or not) for
the facing of the final loss.

AVOIDING PAIN

It is now a well-established truism of death and dying studies that
modern Western culture is a "death-denying culture."[2] This means
that it is a general feature of our culture that the reality of death is

denied, softened, repressed, or avoided wherever possible. "Death" has become the modern taboo.[3] Critics cite our use of death-denying language, such as "passed on" instead of "died," "memorial parks" instead of "cemeteries," or even "wasted" (in the language of gangs) instead of "killed." They point out that the "mortician's art" is based on the modern desire to make the deceased look as if still alive, as if "nothing significant" has happened. In addition, the place of death has changed over the years from the home, where its reality would be witnessed by all, even our children, to the hospital, where death is controlled, sanitized, and isolated from the real world. Modern Americans, lured by the promises of technology, dream that death can be cheated by the latest developments in medicine or the wonders of cryonics.

I suggest that this cultural trend is broader than death denying . . . it is also grief denying. We deny, discourage, suppress the open expression of grief feelings, i.e., mourning. This observation is especially apparent in contrast to less developed societies or to our own society prior to the last century. Philippe Aries, a historian of death in Western civilization, argues that some form of mourning has always been mandatory in human societies until the last century. He writes:

> Only in the twentieth century has it [mourning] been forbidden. The situation was reversed in a single generation: what was always commanded by individual conscience, or the general will, is now rejected.[4]

In contrast to the past, today we have very few grief rituals or prescribed customs for mourning, thus in some ways making grieving more difficult. Today, mourning is expected to be controlled, dignified, and above all, brief. And if one cannot be "controlled, dignified, and brief," then one is expected to take one's "problem" to a psychotherapist, where at the very least it can be handled in private.

This trend toward the denial of grieving is part of a larger pattern in our culture, of course, toward the avoidance of all kinds of pain—physical, psychological, and/or social. The culture emphasizes instant relief from pain or any discomfort. The culture, through its multibillion-dollar advertisement industry promotes instant gratification. We are encouraged, night after night, to medicate pain, mask negative feelings, and flee from sorrow. The result of this conditioning is that we all have lower and lower tolerances for pain, at least compared to our forebears. The traditional virtue "long suffering" or even ordinary "patience" is in short supply among modern, secular Westerners.[5]

When we consider grief sufferers in this cultural context, it is difficult to convince them to fully enter their grieving. It is difficult to tell them that the "only way out is through." They would rather medicate their grief, avoid it, keep it brief. The result is that we have a literal epidemic of unresolved grief in our population. Nobody grieves. Nobody knows how to grieve. Nobody knows the art of suffering well.

LEARNING TO SUFFER WELL

The passion, death, and eventual resurrection of Jesus Christ can be understood as a paradigm for how we are to deal with loss, sorrow, and faith in later life.

If we view Jesus' death and resurrection as a unified process, we immediately notice the importance of the sequential order of the events. Jesus had to die in order to live anew. He could not do the reverse: be glorified now and suffer later. He had to lose in order to gain. That is the necessary order of events. In a similar way we face the same succession of events every time we face a loss in later life. We lose . . . we suffer . . . then we find new life. We might wish to reverse the order. Denial is a way of trying to reverse the order of these events, trying to avoid the loss, trying to "let the cup pass." If we do attempt to avoid grieving, we truncate the normal sequential order, and end up "losing life" (see Mt 16:25). What a strange paradox!

Indeed, something about life, particularly life in the later years, suggests that at times we must lose in order to gain. We must let go in order to find. We must let go of something old in order to receive something new. When losses emerge in our lives, our first impulse is not to let go, but to save, to control, to cling. Yet, it is precisely by doing so that we cut ourselves off from life. Only by losing, by grieving, by letting go, will we find new life. It is indeed a paradox.

Suffering then becomes a necessary part of the death and resurrection experience. Jesus' passion was a necessary part of his death and resurrection. He had to go "through" it. Similarly, our suffering is a necessary part of our dying and rising. We cannot find new life unless we are willing to enter our suffering. For us that suffering means grieving. We cannot move on to a new life stage unless we grieve, fully and completely. Grieving is emotional suffering. It is the necessary suffering that allows us to let go of the past. It is the emotional process that gradually enables us to withdraw our energy from that which is now dead. Obviously, if we cannot do this, we cannot live again.

FAITH AS THE TRUST

The question might legitimately be asked then, "How are we able to embrace grief work?" Grief hurts. What enables us to suffer well?

The Gospel stories tell us very directly that Jesus suffered, that his sufferings were real and necessary. Yet, the Garden of Gethsemane story is also a story of great faith. Jesus had a faith that sustained him and strengthened him in spite of his fears, his doubts, and the anticipatory grief he was experiencing.[6] Faith sustained Jesus and somehow enabled him to enter and eventually transcend his loss.

Faith as trust refers to our trusting attitude toward God. Trust is largely an attitude, a precognitive stance toward God, in fact toward life in general.[7] We do not think our way into trust, although thinking can help. It is more automatic, more feeling oriented, and in fact more universal than thinking would allow. It is human to trust. Faith as trust manifests itself as a trusting attitude toward life, toward others, toward oneself, toward the providential events of life. Faith as trust allows us to enter life in all of its fullness with an experiential confidence that "it is good" (Gen 1:25, 31).

When we experience a loss or first become aware of a loss process, and especially if that loss is unwelcomed or unexpected, our trust is momentarily shattered. Momentarily life seems very distrustful, unpredictable, and malevolent. Our impulse is to hide, to avoid, to deny. There is a powerful temptation to avoid pain and cling, however irrationally, to that which is lost. There is also a growth impulse, an urge to embrace it, to let go and to cry. The forces of avoidance and the forces of growth vie to determine our "decision." Trust battles with distrust. If we can mobilize our sense of trust, perhaps because we have a prior history of successful trust experiences, then we can more easily commence our necessary grief work. Conversely, if distrust prevails, perhaps because we have a prior history of unfinished or distrust experiences, then we would to rather cling to the past, hide from our pain, and avoid the necessary grief work before us.

Benjamin couldn't cry. He mother was dying of cancer in a nearby nursing home—a slow, lingering, prolonged process. He couldn't sleep at night. He was nervous all day. He couldn't concentrate on his work. He sought me out for advice. Benjamin was very close to his mother. She had been his confidante, friend, and motivator even well into his adult years. Her death would be a major loss/change in his life. With my prodding, Benjamin would get close to tears. His eyes would fill up. His lip would quiver—but he couldn't let go. "Come on, Ben," I would urge him. "Let it out. Let it go. I know your pain is great."

"It's too difficult, Doctor. I'm afraid to break down in front of people. I know I need to cry, but it's not my style. That's one of the things my mother always told us kids, you know. Don't show people your emotions; don't show them where you're vulnerable."

"It's a real double bind for you, then," I said. "You want to cry over your mother's imminent death; you love her very much; but you are also bound by her instructions not to cry over her. It would be showing disloyalty to her to cry over her."

"Emotions are troublesome in our family. It goes back to when my people were slaves. You didn't show the white man your weaknesses. They'd get you into trouble. My mother knows I love her. I don't need to cry over her now to prove anything."

"But you're hurting, Ben, and when we hurt, it's often helpful to cry," I observed.

"As I said, emotions are troublesome. They get out of control, overwhelm you with passion or anguish. I prefer to stay in charge of my emotions. It's safer that way."

"I hope that when and where you do feel safe, you might relax and allow yourself some grief, expressed and shared in your own way. I think you will feel a whole lot better."

Benjamin's mother died a few days after this conversation, and he went through the funeral largely self-controlled. I suspect that he let down some in private, but he certainly did not enter the process, and he continued to be bothered by physical symptoms for months after his mother's death. Benjamin had a choice between allowing himself tears or holding them back. It was not entirely a free choice. Cultural and family issues limited his freedom to respond other than in a controlled manner. Perhaps if Benjamin had a more prolonged therapeutic relationship, one in which he could feel safe, he might have shared more of his pain. Unfortunately, that option was not available to us.

The choice of whether to cry or not is as simple and as universal as all that. Each time we deal with a loss, we "face a choice," says Paul Tournier, "a choice between facing reality and evasion."[8] We encounter the same choice over and over again. On the surface it is a choice between whether to grieve or not, but at a deeper level it is a choice whether to grow or not.

FAITH IS LETTING GO

Faith is not experienced in isolation. We are all relational creatures and our faith is either supported or undermined by our closest relationships. Others who have faith when we do not can facilitate our faith. In a real sense we borrow their faith for a while. The importance of others is especially crucial in matters of loss, when our normally adequate faith might feel very inadequate. Loved ones who have faith, or a community of faith can facilitate our grieving, if our faith is momentarily shaky. Those loved ones, however, have to be willing to be engaged with us in our sorrow and theirs.

The movie, *Ordinary People*, based on the novel by Judith Guest, is a powerful study of abnormal grief and the critical role others play in facilitating or blocking grief.[9] Conrad is the younger of two teenage sons of well-to-do parents, Calvin and Beth. The oldest son Buck, who was successful at almost everything he did and who appears to be his parents' favorite, died in a boating accident. Conrad was also involved in the boating accident, but managed to survive. Soon thereafter Conrad attempts suicide and is briefly hospitalized. Conrad still cannot grieve, however, and is haunted by flashbacks and nightmares. He also shows a lack of appetite, preoccupation, irritability, and continuing depression—all of which are the classic symptoms of a stuck grief process. As we gain a broader picture of what this family has endured in the death of Buck, we are impressed by how little they talk about Buck, the accident, or for that matter, anything meaningful. Conrad complains, "We don't connect." What becomes clear is that the whole family, particularly Conrad's mother, Beth, is denying the loss, refusing to grieve, and trying wherever possible to "escape" from the scene both emotionally and physically. Conrad needs to grieve, but he has no social support for it.

Conrad enters regular therapy with Dr. Berger, a local psychiatrist, who helps him begin to feel again. Here we see Conrad struggling with his own inner war between denial and grieving. Part of him wants to feel again and part of him flees from the tremendous pain therein. In one particularly powerful scene, Conrad has just learned that a friend from the hospital has killed herself, news that throws him into an emotional upheaval and places him on the edge of attempting to take his own life again. During an emergency session with his therapist, the conversation goes something like this.

"Feelings are scary," says Dr. Berger. "Sometimes they're painful. If you can't feel pain, you are not going to feel anything else, either. You're alive, and don't tell me you don't feel that."

"It doesn't feel good," responds Conrad.

"It is good—believe me," Berger affirms.

"How do you know?" the boy asks.

"Because I'm your friend."

"I don't know what I would have done if you hadn't been here," says Conrad. "Are you really my friend?"

"I am. Count on it."

In that instant Conrad lets go, embraces his newfound friend and weeps deeply. This is the grief that Conrad had held back for these many months. This is the pain that never came out at the funeral, the pain that was turned inward as depression.

In that moment, Conrad exercised his faith. He made a "leap of faith." He trusted. Conrad entered that scary world of feelings. He trusted his feeling . . . his emotional process. He entered his pain for the first time. Then, and only then, did he begin to heal.

IDOLATRY AND AVOIDING GRIEF

Some people have little faith as trust, and thus, for them grieving is difficult. They find it difficult to experience their feelings, fearing that the feelings will overwhelm them, that nothing or no one will sustain them, and that the process will have no resolution. Such people, as noted in earlier chapters, tend to cling to various defense mechanisms, the most common being denial, as desperate means of trying to control the pain within. Generally, the greater the pain within, the greater the need to try to control, the more rigid or extreme the defense mechanism.

Going back to the movie for a moment, consider Conrad's mother, Beth, who is an example of someone who chose not to grieve. Her style was to avoid pain and strive to cover up anything messy or unpleasant—a decision which obviously damaged Conrad and eventually her marriage. Focus just on her functioning. Do you see anything familiar? She cannot love. She cannot give. She is emotionally aloof. Her interest is in keeping life orderly, pleasant, and pretty. The house must be clean. No one must know about the family secrets. She refuses to allow a pet dog (which would be both messy and giving). She is unable to return love, even when Conrad becomes healed enough to embrace her. Gradually we see how empty her life really is. We see clearly that by trying "to save her life" she is therefore "losing her life."

I argue that if we look at this "living human document" theologically, we would see a woman caught in idolatry. Beth has little faith in God or in anything else that could have encouraged her grief or sustained her in sorrow. Not trusting in this God, she flees from her pain. But where else did she put her faith? What becomes her god? She creates an idol called control, and as long as she worships at this altar it gives her happiness (of sorts). Control becomes her raison d'etre, her identity, and her value system. What becomes increasingly clear to her husband is that she cannot change. She is trapped, imprisoned, maybe even a slave. She ceased to grow spiritually when she refused to grieve.

In the absence of genuine faith, we humans do tend to create our own idols that become particularly potent in times of loss, that enslave us and block us from grieving and thereby growing into new life.

SUCCESSFUL AGING

In the literature on aging, considerable attention is given to the topic of successful aging. It continues to fascinate those who study the psychology of aging, why most people seem to decline mentally, psychologically, and socially in the later years of life, while others seem to grow and expand mentally, psychologically, and socially. Various researchers have attempted to describe what they consider to be optimum aging.[10] Of course, everyone ages slightly differently, but in general what are the characteristics of personality or behavior that enable one to age well, in full mental and spiritual health?

In a textbook on this topic, *Aging and Mental Health,* the authors, Robert N. Butler and Myrna I. Lewis say this about successful aging:

> . . . it is imperative that old people continue to develop and change in flexible manner if health is to be promoted and maintained. Failure of adaptation at any age or under any circumstances can result in physical or emotional illness.[11]

The key phrase is "change in a flexible manner." One of the key psychological ingredients for success in aging is the ability to adapt to change, to be emotionally and mentally flexible. This is so because, in the words of these same authors:

> Loss is a predominant theme in the emotional experience of elderly people . . . losses in every aspect of late life compel the elderly to expend enormous amounts of physical and emotional energy in grieving and resolving grief, adapting to the changes that result from loss, and recovering from the stresses inherent in these processes.[12]

If loss is such a "predominant theme" in the later years, and if emotional "flexibility" and the ability to adapt are such vital ingredients, what are the dynamics that allow people to pass though repeated losses and remain emotionally flexible?

In his book *Ageless Body, Timeless Mind,* Deepak Chopra addresses this same question, "What psychological traits constitute successful aging?" After reviewing the research, particularly of

Flanders Dunbar's work with centenarians, he identifies "psychological adaptability" as the chief trait. He defines adaptability as "freedom from conditioned response." He continues:

> To remain open to change, to accept the new and welcome the unknown, is a choice that involves definite personal skills; for left to inertia, the mind tends to reinforce its old habits and increasingly to fall prey to its conditioning.[13]

Chopra goes so far as to present an Adaptability Questionnaire that might be used to measure the strength of one's psychological adaptability, and by implication, how well one might age.

Robert C. Peck, whose work I have referred to earlier in this book, has come to similar conclusions about the importance of psychological adaptability or "flexibility."[14] He argues that people who are capable of being psychologically flexible are better able to weather the inevitable losses of the second half of life, in contrast to the people who cannot be flexible, and become increasingly "impoverished" as they age. As you will recall, I suggested that Peck's definition of cathectic flexibility sounded much like the ability to do successful grief work.

One of the stereotypes of old age is mental rigidity. We tend to think of elderly people as conservative, as persons who resist new ideas, who cannot change, who are inflexible and who are "stuck in their ways." This view is a stereotype and a dangerous one in the sense that it can easily become prescriptive in nature, not just descriptive.

In this regard, another developmental task of the middle years, according to Peck, is to develop mental flexibility rather than mental rigidity. He notes that adults who maintain or learn mental flexibility are able to learn "to master their experiences, achieve a degree of detached perspective on them, and make use of them as *provisional* guides to the solution of new issues."[15] In contrast, other adults who drift toward mental rigidity seem to become "dominated" by their experiences. They take "the patterns of events and actions which they happen to have encountered, as a set of fixed inflexible rules"[16] which must govern all of their subsequent behavior and thinking. If an older adult is to age well, he or she must master this developmental task of learning to be mentally flexible. Far too many adults tend to grow increasingly set in their ways and closed minded with each passing year.

Why might older people become mentally rigid? Is it an innate tendency of the advancing years or is it a reaction to something else? I suggest that it might be the latter. Increased rigidity might be understood as part of the dynamics of defense mechanisms. Instead of dealing with our feelings of grief, we deny the feelings. We run from them in the opposite direction, toward greater rigidity, a greater sense of control in the face of what seems to be uncontrollable. The psychological term for this is reaction formation. The theological term is idolatry.

Mental rigidity can be understood, simply put, as a reaction to ungrieved losses, to unfaced feelings of sadness and anxiety. Mental flexibility, as in the case of emotional flexibility, is possible only when we grieve our losses. If we want to age well, we need to master the developmental tasks surrounding emotional flexibility and mental flexibility. In short, we need to learn to grieve, to adapt to change and be emotionally and mentally flexible. This is one of the traits of those who age successfully.

FAITH AND AGING WELL

Since losses are such a major part of life in the later years, people who wish to age successfully need to be able to grieve naturally and easily and completely. That assignment is easier said than done. I have observed that most people don't seem to grieve easily or completely, an observation which I think accounts for so much mental, psychological, and social decline in later life. Most older people are just overwhelmed by the cumulative nature of loss and eventually give up in despair.

Yet, some rare people seem to suffer well, seem to rebound from one loss after another. They do not have fewer troubles than the rest of us. No, they have their share of sufferings, maybe even more than most, but they still seem to appreciate life and look forward to living. They seem to have a deep acceptance of life or faith in life's goodness that sustains them and carries them through all of life's sorrows. According to Erikson and others, most of us do not acquire this acceptance until late in life.[17] Perhaps these rare people who seem to age so well have learned acceptance much sooner than the rest of us.

Perhaps they are what Erikson called homo religious, people who have made "the integrity crisis . . . a lifelong and chronic crisis."[18]

Because of this deep acceptance of the inevitability of loss, persons who age successfully have the ability to suffer well. They accept the inevitability of loss in later life. They know that they have no choice about that. But they do know that they have a choice about how they respond to loss. They choose to cry, they choose to suffer deeply, and they also choose to love again . . . and again . . . and again. It is as if they continue to believe that "life is good" no matter how tragic or painful life becomes at times. As a result they continue to care, to grow, and to rise above their sufferings. They continue to go forth joyfully.

All this is made possible, in part, because of their faith, understood as trust. Faith enables them to embrace their pain, to fully experience their grief feelings, and thus, to swiftly pass through the transition, reinvesting themselves in new attachments and in a new stage of life. Through faith, their losses have been transformed into transition, new life has emerged out of old, resurrection has followed death. Thus these rare people now come to the end of their lives with a measure of assurance that the same God who brought them through all of life's previous losses will also walk with them through this final loss, together into the world beyond.

Notes

Preface

R. Scott Sullender, *Grief and Growth: Pastoral Resources for Emotional and Spiritual Growth* (Mahwah, NJ: Paulist Press, 1985).

Chapter 1

1. The idea of varying degrees of denial was introduced to me in Avery D. Weisman, *On Dying and Denying: A Psychiatric Study of Terminality* (New York: Behavioral, 1972). Another word for this type of denial is repression.

2. Another word for this type of denial is repression.

3. In fact, Joan Guntzelman has suggested just such a scheme of grief's stages, based on the three levels of denial described here. Stage One is "acknowledging what has been lost," Stage Two is "express" feelings, and Stage Three is "choosing to change the things that keep us tied to the lost object." See Joan Guntzelman's *Blessed Grieving* (Winona, MN: Christian Brothers Publications, 1994), p. 16.

4. In extreme forms, idealization becomes idolization. The two words have come to mean almost the same thing. This will be discussed more fully in Chapter 2.

5. C. S. Lewis uses the image of a journey to describe the grief process in his story of his own conjugal bereavement. See *A Grief Observed* (London: Faber and Faber, 1961).

6. This understanding of grief, as a function of attachment "instincts," is associated with John Bowley. See *The Making and Breaking of Affectional Bonds* (London: Tavistock Publications, 1979).

7. This is a phrase and philosophy that is associated with Viktor E. Frankl and his school of psychotherapy called "logotherapy." See *Man's Search for Meaning: An Introduction to Logotherapy* (Boston: Beacon Press, 1962).

8. This is due to a combination of factors: the preferred age differential between men and women, the shorter life span of men compared to women, as well as individual factors.

Chapter 2

1. Jacques Ellul, *The Humiliation of the Word* (Grand Rapids: William B. Eerdmans, 1985), p. 93.

2. This is why the Christian message is so unique. In Christ, Christians claim to see God for the first time. God has taken human form precisely so he can be visible to us.

3. See R. M. Lieberf, J. M. Neale, and E. S. Davidson, *The Early Window: Effects of Television on Children and Youth* (New York: Pergamon, 1973).

4. Behavioral psychology tells us that sometimes the occasional reinforcer is more effective than a constant reinforcer.

5. See Merle R. Jordan, *Taking on the Gods: The Task of the Pastoral Counselor* (Nashville: Abingdon, 1986).

6. For the most part, I have tried to avoid sexist language. In referring to God, however, I have used capitalized masculine pronouns. I certainly do not mean to imply a masculine nature to God.

7. Abnormal grief does not have to be characterized by just sorrow. Undue bitterness, depression, or guilt can also be a sign of an unfinished grief process.

8. The last chapter of this book will offer a more extensive discussion of the role of faith in grief and successful aging in the later years.

Chapter 3

1. Leo Missinne, gerontologist from the University of Nebraska, made the remark in a lecture given at Pilgrim Place, Claremont, August 8, 1986.

2. I was first introduced to the term "marker event" in Bernice L. Neugarten's "Adult Personality: A Developmental View," *Human Development*, IX (1965), pp. 61-73.

3. The only socially prescribed marker event in later life is perhaps retirement, but even here there are few commonly accepted rituals. This will be discussed further in Chapter 6.

4. This is especially so for men, who use their work as "an organizing principle" to talk about their adult life stages. See Daniel J. Levinson, *The Seasons of a Man's Life* (New York: Ballantine Books, 1976).

5. The work experience of women is often much different from that of men. Many women are just beginning a career in midlife, instead of plateauing out in one. This is discussed more fully in later chapters. For the moment I just want to make the point that wrestling with career choices in later life is often a disguised way of wrestling with the loss of youth.

6. Judith Viorst, *Necessary Losses* (New York: Simon and Schuster, 1986), p. 269.

7. This observation was first reported in print, in Bernice L. Neugarten, "Adaptation and the Life Cycle," in Nancy K. Schlossberg, Alan D. Entine, editors, *Counseling Adults* (Monterey, CA: Brooks/Cole, 1977), p. 39.

8. "Eschatology" is the branch of theology that studies "the last things," the final end of history. The term is used here as an existential or clinical version of the general concept.

9. Daniel J. Levinson, *The Seasons of a Man's Life*, p. 217.

10. Phillip L. Berman and Connie Goldman, editors, *The Ageless Spirit* (New York: Ballantine Books, 1992), p. 5.

11. Bernice L. Neugarten has done considerable work on the role of social norms in influencing when we complete certain life cycle events. She found that when people complete major developmental tasks is partly based on when they are expected to do so. See "Age Norms, Age Constraints and Adult Socialization," *American Journal of Sociology*, LXX (1965), pp. 710-717.

12. Alex Comfort, *A Good Age* (New York: Crown, 1976), p. 35.

13. Robert W. McClellan in his book, *Claiming the Frontier: Ministry and Older People* (Los Angeles: University of Southern California, 1977) has introduced the term "gerontophobia," which is the "fear of aging." McClellan says this fear is a product of the collective denial of our own aging.

14. Perhaps one could argue that age sixty-five, set by the federal government, is the age at which one is considered legally old. Psychologically some people feel old at forty; others don't consider themselves old until they are seventy-five. The meaning of "old" is also influenced by social norms.

15. Daniel J. Levinson, *The Seasons of a Man's Life*, p. 210.

16. William M. Clements, *Care and Counseling of the Aging* (Philadelphia: Fortress Press, 1979), p. 19. An interesting discussion of the whole low-high-low model of aging may be found on pp. 19-22.

17. Charles E. Curran, "Aging: A Theological Perspective," in Carol LeFevre and Perry LeFevre, *Aging and the Human Spirit: A Reader in Religion and Gerontology*, Second Edition (Chicago: Exploration Press, 1981), p. 74.

18. Rabbi Abraham J. Herchel first introduced me to this image. He uses it in his "Older Person and the Family in the Perspective of Jewish Tradition," in Carol LeFevre and Perry LeFevre's, *Aging and the Human Spirit*, pp. 35-44.

19. See Paul Tournier, *Learn to Grow Old* (New York: Harper and Row, 1972).

20. Ibid., pp. 184-185.

21. See Elisabeth Kübler-Ross, *On Death and Dying* (New York: Macmillan, 1969).

22. Eugene C. Bianchi, *Aging As a Spiritual Journey* (New York: Crossroad, 1982), p. 16.

Chapter 4

1. Reflect for a moment: What is the hidden idol being worshiped here?

2. Roger L. Gould, *Transformations: Growth and Change in the Adult Life* (New York: Simon and Schuster, 1978), p. 225.

3. Many of the problems encountered by families with adolescents can be summarized as poor timing: either the child wants more independence than the parents are ready to give or the parents give the child more freedom than the teenager is ready to handle. In both cases conflicts emerge. Effective parenting, then, assumes a readiness to let go in apportion to the child's level of responsibility.

4. Herbert Anderson, *The Family and Pastoral Care* (Philadelphia: Fortress Press, 1984), pp. 63-64.

5. Reviewing photographs or family albums is often a good way to begin grief work with an individual or a family.

6. The ritual that comes closest to being a marker event for the loss of family is the wedding of one of the children. Often in the midst of this ritual, the parents grieve the loss of their daughter or son and in a larger sense the loss of their family. Clergy would do well to be aware of this dimension of the wedding ceremony.

7. You can see clearly how the loss of family and the loss of youth can be entangled in some adults. Actually, all of these losses are interrelated and can mutually reinforce or block another's grief.

8. The loss of a home is often associated with the loss of family. Many post-parenting couples, for example, relocate to smaller, more manageable quarters after the children leave home.

9. Thomas Bradley Robb, *The Bonus Years: Foundations for Ministry with Older Persons* (Valley Forge: The Judson Press, 1968), p. 64.

10. Robert C. Peck, "Psychological Developments in the Second Half of Life," in Bernice L. Neugarten, editor, *Middle Age and Aging* (Chicago: University of Chicago Press, 1968), p. 89.

11. Reul L. Howe first used the phrase "creative years" to describe this stage of life in the 1950s. See his *Creative Years* (Greenwich, CT: Seabury Press, 1959).

12. It is not just the strength of the attachment that makes grief more difficult and complex, but also the availability and presence of other psychosocial resources, i.e., the presence and quality of the marital dyad, the availability of midlife vocational options, the absence of codependent traits and the relative psychological stability of the individual.

13. See Bernice L. Neugarten, "Adaptation and Life Cycle," in *Counseling Adults*, pp. 34-46.

14. A good question to ask is "Who owns this problem?" If it is the adult child that owns the problem, the parents' roles are those of listener and, when asked, advice giver.

15. Daniel Levinson's version of this same dynamic is captured in the word "legacy." He says that the midlife man is concerned with legacy and that this concern can take many forms, including children, passing on material possessions, and/or creating work that will transcend him. See Daniel J. Levinson, *The Seasons of a Man's Life* (New York: Ballantine Books, 1976, pp. 219ff).

16. See Don S. Browning, *Generative Man: Psychoanalytic Perspectives* (Philadelphia: Westminster Press, 1973).

Chapter 5

1. The source of these figures is the U.S. Bureau of the Census as reported in Ken Dychtwald and Joe Flower, *Age Wave: How the Most Important Trend of Our Time Will Change Your Future* (New York: Bantam Books, 1990), p. 6.

2. In 1995, 12.8 percent of the U.S. population was age 65 or older. By year 2030 it is projected to be 15.1 percent and by year 2050, 24.8 percent. Source is Bureau of the Census, United States Department of Commerce, as reported in *The World Almanac and Book of Facts* (New York: World Almanac Books, 1998), p. 366.

3. See Judith Treas, "Intergenerational Families and Social Change," in Pauline K. Ragan, editor, *Aging Parents* (Los Angeles: University of Southern California Press, 1979), pp. 58-65.

4. In fact, as the life span continues to lengthen, it may become more and more common for adult children to still be caring for an aged parent even after they themselves have entered retirement. Bernice L. Neugarten, for example, now says that we have to talk about the middle generations in the plural, and conceive of a family structure of four and five generations. See her article, "The Middle Generations," in *Aging Parents*, pp. 258-266.

5. The actual research on this point shows mixed results. Some studies suggest that most older Americans live within one hour of at least one of their children. Other studies have indicated that fifty percent of older Americans have no living relative close at hand. For a summary of this material, see James A. Peterson's article, "The Relationships of Middle-Aged Children and Their Parents," in *Aging Parents*, pp. 27-36.

6. Dependency in old age is actually related more to declining mental and physical functioning than to any particular age. The so-called "young old" are still very independent and often see their children's caring as premature.

7. Dr. Missinne made this observation in the "Adventure in Aging Workshop" at Pilgrim Place, Claremont, California, on August 8, 1986.

8. Occasionally we can even experience some anger/frustration that our ailing parent doesn't die sooner and "get it over with," so we can got on with our lives. This is a difficult type of anger to manage.

9. The most obvious helpful procedure is for family members to discuss such issues ahead of time and perhaps make out a living will.

10. Edward Myers, *When Parents Die: A Guide for Adults* (New York: Viking Penguin, 1986), p. 5.

11. Ira S. Hirschfield and Helen Dennis, "Perspectives," in *Aging Parents,* p. 13.

12. Smiley Blanton, *Now or Never: The Promise of the Middle Years* (Carmel, New York: Guideposts Associates, 1959), p. 236. Dr. Blanton, along with Reverend Norman Vincent Peale, founded the Institute for Religion and Health in New York City.

13. Many grieving people, "act out" their guilt through the funeral and its related trappings. The funeral industry has been severely criticized over the years for playing on this inevitable guilt in the survivor's sorrow. Yet, in another sense I have witnessed occasions when an ostentatious funeral actually helped release a grieving adult child from a plaguing sense of guilt. Perhaps it was so because he or she could now do something concrete to make it up to Mom or Dad. Forgiveness can be secured in different ways.

14. Those are difficult decisions. Fortunately there are many fine books being written on this subject of medical ethics these days. In addition many hospitals have clinically trained chaplains or pastoral counselors who can assist you with ethical decisions.

15. Parents and grandparents are typically the keepers of the family history. In recent years there has been more interest among families in recording the family

histories before parents die. In addition to its historical value, it is a valuable experience in anticipatory grieving.

16. However, more commonly, the death of our last parent is occurring later and later in our life cycle. We can be well into retirement and the later stages of our life cycle before our last parent dies. In such cases, the sense of eschatology spoken of in this paragraph, usually associated with the midlife crisis, is less intense.

Chapter 6

1. Mandatory retirement is now opposed by several lobbying groups as an example of ageism, discrimination based on one's age, in contrast to how it was received when it was initially instituted.

2. For a summary of this research, see Carl Eisdorfer, "Adaption to Loss of Work," in F. Carp, editor, *Retirement* (New York: Human Science Press, 1972).

3. Douglas C. Kimmel, *Adulthood and Aging*, Third Edition (New York: Wiley and Sons, 1990), p. 305.

4. Ibid., p. 314.

5. It is an interesting contradiction that while the mandatory retirement age has gone up to age seventy, the average age of retirement has actually dropped to its current 58.6 years.

6. Eugene A. Friedmann and Robert J. Havighurst, *The Meaning of Work and Retirement* (Chicago: University of Chicago Press, 1954).

7. See Robert J. Havighurst, "Life Style and Leisure Patterns," in Richard A. Kalish, editor, *The Later Years* (Monterey, CA: Brooks/Cole, 1977), pp. 147-156.

8. For example, see I. H. Simpson, K. W. Black, and J. C. McKinney, "Work and Retirement," in I. H. Simpson and J. C. McKinney, editors, *Social Aspects of Aging* (Durham: Duke University Press, 1966), pp. 45-54.

9. Bert Hayship Jr. and Paul E. Panek, *Adult Development and Aging* (San Francisco: Harper and Row, 1989), p. 416.

10. Writers have noted another interesting trend—the long-term shift from self-employed to working for others. This has occurred in the last 100 years, and has made retirement easier.Ibid., pp. 410-411.

11. Friedmann and Havighurst, *The Meaning of Work and Retirement*, p. 189.

12. This is a point of view that I do not entirely agree with, and I will say more about it later.

13. See Richard E. Leakey, *Origins* (New York: E.P. Dutton, 1977), pp. 207-238.

14. In fact, Robert N. Bellah's *Habits of the Heart: Individualism and Commitment in American Life* (Berkeley:University of California Press, 1985) suggests that themes of competition, individualism, and privatization of life are becoming more (not less) pronounced in American culture as we approach the twenty-first century.

15. This conclusion was noted in Chapter 3 too. See Daniel J. Levinson, *The Seasons of a Man's Life* (New York: Ballantine Books, 1976).

16. Eugene C. Bianchi, *Aging As a Spiritual Journey* (New York: Crossroad, 1982), p. 162.

17. Henri J. M. Nouwen and Walter J. Gaffney, *Aging: The Fulfillment of Life* (New York: Doubleday, 1976), p. 33.

18. My comments have been informed by Dorothee Soelle's *To Work and to Love* (Philadelphia: Fortress Press, 1984) which is a provocative discussion of this topic and other related issues.

19. Admittedly, this is an oversimplification of these two important theological concepts about work. However, it is often these simplified versions that shape culture so decisively.

20. See Richard N. Bolles, *The Three Boxes of Life* (Berkeley: Ten Speed Press, 1981).

21. The problem of retirement is not, as some scholars suggest, a problem of leisure, how to learn to be better consumers and content with leisure activities. Each stage of life should include a blending of work and play. Therefore retirement should not be thought of as the absence of work, but as the time for what Paul Tournier calls a "Second Career," for a type of work that is both work and play, two forms of creative self-expression. See Paul Tournier, *Learn to Grow Old* (New York: Harper, 1972), p. 123

22. Evelyn Eaton Whitehead and James D. Whitehead, "Retirement," in William M. Clements, editor, *Ministry with the Aging: Design, Challenges, Foundations* (New York: Harper and Row, 1981), p. 133.

23. Thomas Bradley Robb, *The Bonus Years: Foundations for Ministry with Older Persons* (Valley Forge: The Judson Press, 1968), p. 96.

Chapter 7

1. See U.S. Bureau of the Census, *Current Population Reports,* Series P. 23, No. 138, "Demographic and Socioeconomic Aspects of Aging in the United States." (Washington, DC: U.S. Government Printing Office, 1984).

2. Robert O. Hansson, Jacqueline H. Remondet, and Marlene Galusha. "Old Age and Widowhood: Issues of Personal Control and Independence," in *Handbook of Bereavement: Theory, Research, and Intervention,* Margaret S. Stroebe, Wolfgang Stroebe, and Robert O. Hansson, editors, (Cambridge, England: Cambridge University Presss, 1993), p. 367.

3. Ibid., p. 374.

4. See Chapter 2 of Colin Murray Parkes, *Bereavement: Studies in Grief in Adult Life* (New York: International Universities Press, 1972).

5. Margaret S. Stroebe and Wolfgang Stroebe, "The Mortality of Bereavement: A Review," in *Handbook of Bereavement: Theory, Research, and Intervention,* p. 194.

6. The research suggests, generally, that unexpected loss is much more difficult to adjust to, and potentially more risky over a broad range of categories, than losses that are gradual in nature.

7. See Robert Jay Lifton, *Death in Life* (New York: Random House, 1967).

8. In 1985, for example, there were 104 million single women over 65 and 2.7 million single men. See "Late-Life Divorce" in Ken Dychtwald and Joe

Flower, *Age Wave: How the Most Important Trend of Our Time Will Change Your Future* (New York: Bantam Books, 1990), p. 215.

9. See Carol M. Anderson and Susan Stewart, with Sona Dimidjian, *Flying Solo: Single Women in Midlife* (New York: W.W. Norton, 1994), p. 81.

10. Mortimer R. Feinberg, Gloria Feinberg and John J. Tarrant, *Leavetaking* (New York: Simon and Schuster, 1978), pp. 239-240.

11. I am drawing on Henri J. M. Nouwen's distinction between care and cure. See his article, "Care and the Elderly," in Carol LeFevre and Perry LeFevre, editors, *Aging and Human Spirit: A Reader in Religion and Gerontology*, Second Edition (Chicago: Exploration Press, 1981), pp. 323-328. I will return to this theme in Chapter 8.

12. "Connectedness," or social support, is a major factor in maintaining physical and mental health in the second half of life and was recently reaffirmed in MacArthur Foundation Study of Aging in America, as summarized in John W. Rowe and Robert L. Kahn, *Successful Aging* (New York: Pantheon Books, 1998).

13. I recognize that there is a popular theory of aging, called the "disengagement theory," associated with Elaine Cumming, that argues that older people do naturally "disengage" from society as they age, and that this is normal. I argue that this is typical, but not necessarily desirable. See Elaine Cumming and William E. Henry, *Growing Old: The Process of Disengagement* (New York: Basic Books, 1961).

14. Eugene C. Bianchi, *Aging As a Spiritual Journey* (New York: Crossroad, 1982), p. 220.

Chapter 8

1. All of the losses discussed in this book are interrelated. One loss may trigger and/or reinforce another loss, which in turn may make us aware of still a third pending loss.

2. Eugene C. Bianchi, *Aging As a Spiritual Journey* (New York: Crossroad, 1982), p. 143.

3. Another way to look at this idolatry theologically is as an ultimate reliance on human effort instead of on God's grace. It is the ultimate form of earning our own salvation. Health worshipers practice this kind of reliance on technology and one's own efforts to "earn" the promised salvation.

4. For a more sophisticated discussion of the interrelationship of health and salvation, see James N. Lapsley, *Salvation and Health: The Interlocking Processes of Life* (Philadelphia: Westminster Press, 1972).

5. "1981 National Ambulatory Medical Care Survey," National Center for Health Statistics, as reported in Karen A. Conner's *Aging America: Issues Facing an Aging Society* (Englewood Cliffs, NJ: Prentice-Hall, 1991).

6. Ibid., p. 88.

7. For fuller discussion of curing versus caring, see Henri J. M. Nouwen and Walter J. Gaffney, *Aging: The Fulfillment of Life* (Garden City, NJ: Image Books, 1976), pp. 89-143.

8. Henri J. M. Nouwen, "Care and the Elderly," in *Aging and Human Spirit,* Second Edition, Carol LeFevre and Perry Le Fevre, editors (Chicago: Exploration Press, 1981), p. 324.

9. See Robert C. Peck, "Psychological Developments in the Second Half of Life," in Bernice L. Neugarten, editor, *Middle Age and Aging* (Chicago: University of Chicago Press, 1968), pp. 88-92.

10. Admittedly it is a paradox: valuing ourselves more as spiritual beings and staying involved in the world. The inner focus and outer focus can and do go together, because at the deepest levels of our souls we are all linked to one another, to the earth, and to God.

11. See Henri J. M. Nouwen, *Aging: The Fulfillment of Life,* p. 33.

Chapter 9

1. She first made this distinction in "Age Groups in American Society and the Rise of the Young-Old," in *Annals of the American Academy of Political and Social Science*, Volume 415, 1974, pp. 187-198.

2. Federal Highway Administration, United States Department of Transportation, as reported in *The World Almanac and Book of Facts*, (New York: World Almanac Books, 1998), p. 214.

3. By eighty-five and older, drivers have more serious injury and fatal accidents per mile driven than teen drivers. "No. 1016. Fatal Motor Vehicle Accidents—National Summary: 1980-1992," in *Statistical Abstracts of the United States*, 114th edition (New York: The Reference Press, Inc. 1994). p. 633.

4. Lewis R. Aiken, *Aging: An Introduction to Gerontology* (Thousand Oaks, CA: Sage, 1995), p. 285.

5. "Old, Alone, and Poor: A Plan for Reducing Poverty Among Elderly People Living Alone." The Commonwealth Fund. As reported in Douglas C. Kimmel, *Adulthood and Aging: An Interdisciplinary, Development View* (New York: Wiley, 1990), p. 481.

6. For an interesting discussion of this issue, see Judith Viorst, *Imperfect Control: Our Lifelong Struggles with Power and Surrender* (New York: Simon and Schuster, 1998).

7. The Serenity Prayer, originally written by Reinhold Niebuhr, has become incorporated into the Alcoholics Anonymous program. The question of control is especially bothersome for people who have addictive disorders. They are often trying to overcontrol their environment, while at the same time, at a another level, they are personally out of control. Although addicts lack self-control, at the base of their disorder is often a desire or an illusion that they can and should control life.

8. "Learned helplessness" is associated with Martin E. Seligman. See *Helplessness* (New York: W. H. Freeman, 1992).

9. The concept of "locus of control" has been around for thirty years or more. More recently, it has been summarized in Herbert M. Lefcourt, *Locus of Control* (New Jersey: Lawrence Erlbaum Associates, 1982).

10. Another similar concept, from the studies of cognition and motivation, is embodied in the term, "self-efficacy," first proposed by Albert Bandura. See Albert Bandura, *Self-Efficacy: The Exercise of Control* (New York: Freeman, 1997).

11. The point that psychological attitudes, i.e., apathy or learned helplessness, can influence the aging process itself, has been made most recently by Deepak Chopra, MD. See *Ageless Body, Timeless Mind: The Quantum Alternative to Growing Old* (New York: Harmony Books, 1993).

12. Ibid., p. 90.

13. I think that this principle has been implied in the "death with dignity" and hospice movement, which try to give the dying person as much control over the process as possible. The ultimate loss of control is death. Yet, even here, if people can maintain some measure of control over their own dying process, it helps them handle it better than if perceived as mere helpless victims.

14. In fact, the study of the human personality tells us that the person who is extremely independent may be overcompensating for an equally strong need for dependence, and vice versa.

Chapter 10

1. The thesis that people grieve as they have lived, or people handle the present loss as they handled the earlier ones, is confirmed in the classic study of retirement (loss of work) by Suzanne Reichard, Florine Livson, and Paul G. Peterson, *Aging and Personality* (New York: Wiley, 1962). They identify five personality types and show how each type typically handles the retirement transition.

2. One of the strongest proponents of death-denying culture is Elisabeth Kübler-Ross. See *On Death and Dying* (New York: Macmillian, 1969). The pioneering book, from a sociological perspective, was Jessica Mitford's *The American Way of Death* (New York: Simon and Schuster, 1963).

3. The use of the phrase, "death as a social taboo," is attributed to Gregory Gorer, who argued that death is the modern taboo, as sex was to the nineteen century. See *Death, Grief, and Mourning* (New York: Doubleday, 1965).

4. Philippe Aries. "Death Inside Out" in the series titled "Eight Centuries of Death in the West," *Hastings Center Studies* (May 1974), Vol. 2, No. 2, p. 10.

5. It is interesting to note that the ability to suffer, usually termed "long suffering" in Scripture, is often listed as one of the results of having mature faith.

6. Faith could thus be understood as a type of courage or as resulting in courage. For a discussion of faith as courage, see Paul Tillich's *Dynamics of Faith* (New York: Harper and Row, 1957).

7. Faith as trust is very close to what Erik Erikson means by "basic trust." For a fuller discussion of this point, see Chapter 9 in my *Grief and Growth* (Mahwah, New Jersey: Paulist Press, 1985), pp. 192-215.

8. Paul Tournier, *Learn to Grow Old* (New York: Harper and Row, 1972), pp. 184-185.

9. It is interesting to note that James W. Fowler also quotes this story, from the book version, in his book *Stages of Faith* (New York: Harper and Row, 1981). We are making different points, but he seems to sense, as I do, that this story is about faith as much as it is about grief. In fact, I suggest that faith and grief are deeply and intricately connected. One cannot grieve well without an implicit faith.

10. For example, see Richard H. Williams and Claudine G. Wirth, *Lives Through the Years: Styles of Life and Successful Aging* (New York: Atherton Press, 1965) or see John W. Rowe and Robert L. Kahn, *Successful Aging* (New York: Pantheon Books, 1998), which summarizes the current scientific research on the subject, with an emphasis on the physical and cognitive dimensions.

11. Robert N. Butler and Myrna I. Lewis, *Aging and Mental Health: Positive Psychosocial Approaches* (Saint Louis, MO: The C.V. Mosby Co., 1973), p. 18.

12. Ibid., p. 29.

13. Deepak Chopra, *Ageless Body, Timeless Mind* (New York: Harmony Books, 1993), p. 73.

14. See Robert C. Peck, "Psychological Developments in the Second Half of Life," in *Middle Age and Aging*. Bernice L. Neugarten, editor (Chicago: University of Chicago Press, 1965), p. 90.

15. Ibid.

16. Ibid.

17. In describing the last developmental crisis of the life cycle, ego integrity versus despair, Erikson defines integrity in this way: "It is the *acceptance* of one's one and only life cycle as something that had to be and that, by necessity, permitted of no substitutions . . . " (emphasis is mine) in *Childhood and Society* (New York: Norton, 1963), p. 268. It is also interesting to note that Elisabeth Kübler-Ross labeled the last stage of the emotional process of terminally ill patients "acceptance." Similar to Erikson, she contrasted acceptance with resignation. Acceptance was more of a positive embracing of life, accepting of loss and what had to be.

18. Erik H. Erikson, *Young Man Luther* (New York: W.W. Norton, 1958), p. 261.

Selected Bibliography

There are many books on aging and grief worth reading. I have tried to select books here that are readable and scholarly and written from an integrated perspective.

Anderson, Herbert and Freda A. Gardner. *Living Alone*. Louisville: Westminster John Knox Press, 1997.

Baum, Gregory, editor. *Work and Religion*. New York: Seabury Press, 1980.

Becker, Arthur H. *Ministry with Older Persons: A Guide for Clergy and Congregations*. Minneapolis: Augsbury Publishing House, 1982.

Bianchi, Eugene C. *Aging As a Spiritual Journey*. New York: Crossroad, 1982.

Capps, Donald. *Life Cycle Theory and Pastoral Care*. Philadelphia: Fortress Press, 1983.

Clements, William M. *Care and Counseling of the Aging*. Philadelphia: Fortress Press, 1979.

_____, editor. *Ministry with the Aging: Design, Challenges, Foundations*. New York: Harper and Row, 1981.

Faber, Heije. *Striking Sails: A Pastoral Psychological View of Growing Older in Our Society*. Translated by Kenneth R. Mitchell. Nashville: Abington Press, 1984.

Fowler, James W. *Stages of Faith*. New York: Harper and Row, 1981.

Hulme, William E. *Vintage Years: Growing Older with Meaning and Hope*. Philadelphia: Westminster Press, 1986.

Kimble, Melvin A. and Susan H. McFadden. *Aging, Spirituality, and Religion: A Handbook*. Philadelphia: Augsburg Fortress, 1995.

Koenig, Harold G. *Aging and God: Spiritual Pathways to Mental Health in Midlife and Later Years*. Binghamton, NY: The Haworth Press, 1994.

Koenig, Harold G. and Andrew J. Weaver. *Pastoral Care of Older Adults*. Philadelphia: Fortress Press, 1998.

LeFevre, Carol and Perry LeFevre. *Aging and the Human Spirit: A Reader in Religion and Gerontology*, Second Edition. Chicago: Exploration Press, 1981.

Lester, Andrew D. and Judith L. Lester. *Understanding Aging Parents*. Philadelphia: Westminster Press, 1980.

Maitland, David J. *Looking Both Ways: A Theology for Midlife*. Atlanta: John Knox Press, 1985.

Mitchell, Kenneth R. and Herbert Anderson. *All Our Losses, All Our Griefs: Resources for Pastoral Care*. Philadelphia: Westminster Press, 1983.

Nouwen, Henri J. M. and Walter J. Gaffney. *Aging: The Fulfillment of Life.* Garden City, NY: Image Books, 1976.

Seeber, James J., editor. *Spiritual Maturity in the Later Years.* Binghamton, NY: The Haworth Press, 1990.

Sullender, R. Scott. *Grief and Growth: Pastoral Resources for Emotional and Spiritual Growth.* Mahwah, NJ: Paulist Press, 1985.

Index

THE HAWORTH PASTORAL PRESS
Pastoral Care, Ministry, and Spirituality
Richard Dayringer, ThD
Senior Editor

LOSSES IN LATER LIFE: A NEW WAY OF WALKING WITH GOD, SECOND EDITION by R. Scott Sullender. "Continues to be a timely and helpful book. There is an empathetic tone throughout, even though the book is a bold challenge to grieve for the sake of growth and maturity and faithfulness. . . . An important book." *Herbert Anderson, PhD, Professor of Pastoral Theology, Catholic Theological Union, Chicago, Illinois*

CARING FOR PEOPLE FROM BIRTH TO DEATH edited by James E. Hightower Jr. "An expertly detailed account of the hopes and hazards folks experience at each stage of their lives. Your empathy will be deepened and your care of people will be highly informed." *Wayne E. Oates, PhD, Professor of Psychiatry Emeritus, School of Medicine, University of Louisville, Kentucky*

HIDDEN ADDICTIONS: A PASTORAL RESPONSE TO THE ABUSE OF LEGAL DRUGS by Bridget Clare McKeever. "This text is a must-read for physicians, pastors, nurses, and counselors. It should be required reading in every seminary and Clinical Pastoral Education program." *Martin C. Helldorfer, DMin, Vice President, Mission, Leadership Development and Corporate Culture, Catholic Health Initiatives—Eastern Region, Pennsylvania*

THE EIGHT MASKS OF MEN: A PRACTICAL GUIDE IN SPIRITUAL GROWTH FOR MEN OF THE CHRISTIAN FAITH by Frederick G. Grosse. "Thoroughly grounded in traditional Christian spirituality and thoughtfully aware of the needs of men in our culture. . . . Close attention could make men's groups once again a vital spiritual force in the church." *Eric O. Springsted, PhD, Chaplain and Professor of Philosophy and Religion, Illinois College, Jacksonville, Illinois*

THE HEART OF PASTORAL COUNSELING: HEALING THROUGH RELATIONSHIP, REVISED EDITION by Richard Dayringer. "Richard Dayringer's revised edition of *The Heart of Pastoral Counseling* is a book for every person's pastor and a pastor's every person." *Glen W. Davidson, Professor, New Mexico Highlands University, Las Vegas, New Mexico*

WHEN LIFE MEETS DEATH: STORIES OF DEATH AND DYING, TRUTH AND COURAGE by Thomas W. Shane. "A kaleidoscope of compassionate, artfully tendered pastoral encounters that evoke in the reader a full range of emotions." *The Rev. Dr. James M. Harper, III, Corporate Director of Clinical Pastoral Education, Health Midwest; Director of Pastoral Care, Baptist Medical Center and Research Medical Center, Kansas City Missouri*

A MEMOIR OF A PASTORAL COUNSELING PRACTICE by Robert L. Menz. "Challenges the reader's belief system. A humorous and abstract book that begs to be read again, and even again." *Richard Dayringer, ThD, Professor and Director, Program in Psychosocial Care, Department of Medical Humanities; Professor and Chief, Division of Behavioral Science, Department of Family and Community Medicine, Southern Illinois University School of Medicine*

Order Your Own Copy of
This Important Book for Your Personal Library!

LOSSES IN LATER LIFE
A New Way of Walking with God, Second Edition

_____ in hardbound at $29.95 (ISBN: 0-7890-0627-8)

_____ in softbound at $19.95 (ISBN: 0-7890-0628-6)

COST OF BOOKS_____

OUTSIDE USA/CANADA/
MEXICO: ADD 20%_____

POSTAGE & HANDLING_____
*(US: $3.00 for first book & $1.25
for each additional book)
Outside US: $4.75 for first book
& $1.75 for each additional book)*

SUBTOTAL_____

IN CANADA: ADD 7% GST_____

STATE TAX_____
*(NY, OH & MN residents, please
add appropriate local sales tax)*

FINAL TOTAL_____
*(If paying in Canadian funds,
convert using the current
exchange rate. UNESCO
coupons welcome.)*

☐ **BILL ME LATER:** ($5 service charge will be added)
(Bill-me option is good on US/Canada/Mexico orders only;
not good to jobbers, wholesalers, or subscription agencies.)

☐ Check here if billing address is different from
shipping address and attach purchase order and
billing address information.

Signature_____

☐ **PAYMENT ENCLOSED: $**_____

☐ **PLEASE CHARGE TO MY CREDIT CARD.**

☐ Visa   ☐ MasterCard   ☐ AmEx   ☐ Discover

Account # _____

Exp. Date _____

Signature _____

Prices in US dollars and subject to change without notice.

NAME _____

INSTITUTION _____

ADDRESS _____

CITY _____

STATE/ZIP _____

COUNTRY _____ COUNTY (NY residents only) _____

TEL _____ FAX _____

E-MAIL_____
May we use your e-mail address for confirmations and other types of information? ☐ Yes   ☐ No

Order From Your Local Bookstore or Directly From
The Haworth Press, Inc.
10 Alice Street, Binghamton, New York 13904-1580 • USA
TELEPHONE: 1-800-HAWORTH (1-800-429-6784) / Outside US/Canada: (607) 722-5857
FAX: 1-800-895-0582 / Outside US/Canada: (607) 772-6362
E-mail: getinfo@haworthpressinc.com
PLEASE PHOTOCOPY THIS FORM FOR YOUR PERSONAL USE.

BOF96